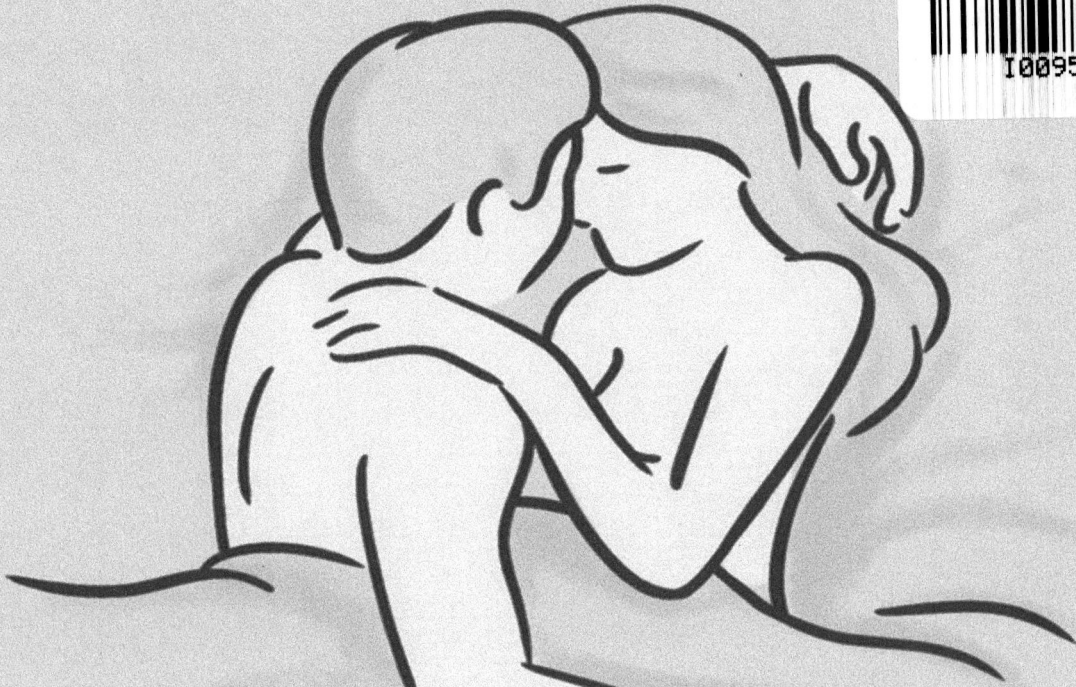

The Ultimate Intimacy Guide for Passionate People

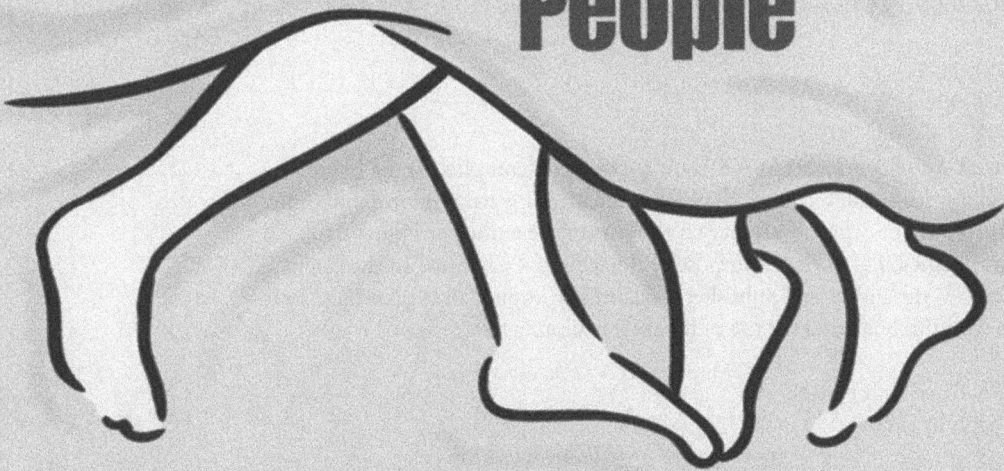

Pillow Book Media Pte. Ltd
Singapore Business Registration 201316808N
©Pillow Book Media 2017

ISBN-10 981-11-2430-2
ISBN-13 978-981-11-2430-3 (pbk)

TYPESET by diacriTech Ptv Ltd
COVER design by Paolo

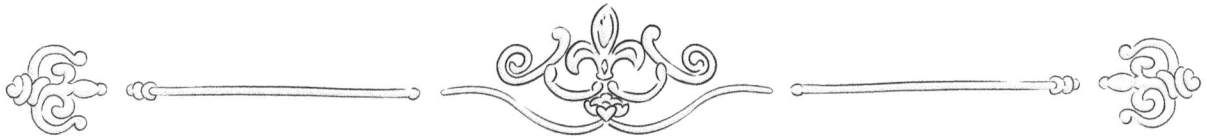

TABLE OF CONTENTS

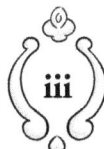

INTRODUCTION

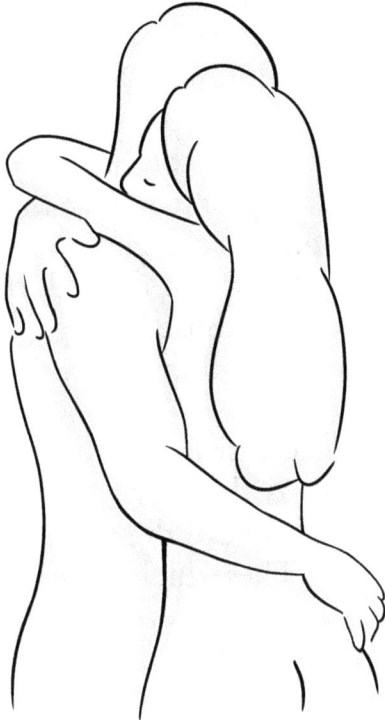

The Ultimate Intimacy Guide for Passionate People is written by Dr. Dawn Michael, to help individuals and couples learn how to work together to create more intimate, loving connections, and improve their sex lives. In her first book *My Husband Won't Have Sex With Me,* Dr. Michael talks about how both men and women have issues with sex and not having the tools they need to enhance the sexual aspect of their relationship. This guidebook is recommended both as a standalone reference, as well as a supplement to her first book, *My Husband Won't Have Sex With Me*.

After 19 years of working with couples, Dr. Michael felt traditional therapeutic tools were inadequate in addressing the sexual issues that many couples were experiencing in their relationships. In fact, most traditional therapeutic approaches focused on diagnosis rather than solutions. Dr. Michael saw the need to develop a guidebook that would enable couples to open up to each other about their sex lives. She understood that for many couples, the little issues in a relationship have the tendency to snowball and become a problem once the intimate connection is gone. Couples could talk for hours about what they were upset about, but when it came down to feelings, it usually boiled down to the lack of intimacy in the relationship along with the skills to communicate those feelings. There is nothing more powerful than the emotions that touch can bring about.

A couple's intimate life can be disrupted by normal everyday issues in addition to larger underlying problems that may never be addressed. Any changes a person experiences in their life also have the potential to affect the quality of sex experienced in the relationship. These include aging, pregnancy, a new job, an illness, negative feelings, past sexual experiences, lack of sex education, just to name a few. Once we can better understand how our body functions sexually, we can show our partner and they too, can do the same. As our physical bodies and our minds mature, so do our sexual mind and body. What someone may have found arousing in their 20s may differ in their later years. Without proper information and guidance regarding the norms concerning age and sexuality, what might initially be a normal sex age-related issue can have the potential to develop into a deeper sexual problem.

Another area of concern is the way a person views sex and intimacy—one's perception of sex could be different from their partners'. Learning how to communicate with each another about sexual issues is crucial for creating more intimacy in the relationship. Intimacy counseling helps couples understand the vital importance of intimacy. Without it, sex can become something bad, uncomfortable, boring, painful, or even unenjoyable.

There are many ways to have intimacy without intercourse. In addition, penetration does not equal sex, it is merely a part of the sexual act that may or may not happen for couples. An individual may be unaware that one need not always engage a particular part of another person's body or perform a particular function, for it to be considered sex. Some people have disabilities or an illness that may prevent them from performing certain sexual acts but that should not prevent anyone from enjoying sexual intimacy with another person.

CASE IN POINT

I had a mature gentleman in his 70s who came to me for help with his sex life. He underwent a successful operation and was treated of his prostate cancer a few years back and this resulted in his inability to achieve or maintain an erection even during masturbation. He was in a relationship and very much wanted to enjoy the sexual experience with his partner. I encouraged him to masturbate even though he was not able to maintain an erection, as I felt that he could still have an orgasm. I specially selected exercises from this guidebook for him to practise and during our next appointment, he was excited to tell me that he was able to have an orgasm and how this was life-changing for him. We then went on to talk about more intimacy exercises he could do with his girlfriend and it was not before long that he was off to a fabulous new sexually fulfilling relationship.

Helping couples understand these basic principles and showing them how to achieve sexual intimacy in other ways can allow for more variety in their sex lives. One of the reasons intimacy counseling works so well is that it is not based on the idea that either party in the relationship needs to be fixed, or one has to change who he/she is.

This is about having new experiences, learning about oneself, reframing ideas surrounding sexuality, healing from past pain, engaging in sex education, empowering oneself with the proper communication tools as well as techniques, and ultimately moving forward in a sex positive direction. Another key aspect of intimacy counseling is teaching couples how to find pleasure in sexual intimacy as well as to have fun in the process. When sex is regarded so seriously that all the pleasure and fun has been taken out of it, it can become a chore or duty instead of a pleasant experience.

Intimacy counseling as opposed to other forms of therapy or psychotherapy, is short-term and solution-based. Couples can work at their own pace and check back if needed for a quick refresher course. Intimacy counseling is proactive and based on the principle of health. As such, individuals need to provide their full sex history so that a counselor can better understand their background, notions about of sex and sexual experiences. This is based on the concept that it takes at least 3 months for one to adjust to a new routine or new idea. As a couple ages, they should always check back on their progress of their sex life as more often than not, we have patterns or comfort zones which can be detrimental to a relationship.

The Ultimate Intimacy Guide for Passionate People addresses the problems that most couples experience at some point in their lives and provides the necessary tools for the couple to work together on their relationship to create better intimacy. When couples can work on their sex lives together and make it more pleasurable, they will feel the connection of true sexual intimacy. In this book, you and your partner will learn how to understand each other and put the joy back into lovemaking. After all, without the connection of the mind and body working together and connecting with another individual, sex is merely a physical act instead of the enjoyment of having connected intimate sex.

Dr. Michael found that by substituting the word 'SEX' with 'INTIMACY', this became a way to help people realize that 'SEX' is not a taboo, but part of what we share with our partner in an intimate way. The problem arises when the 'INTIMACY' is taken out of 'SEX', leaving a void that is hard to describe for many couples and even more difficult to fix in the absence of proper tools.

[ONE]

THE CONCEPT OF FAMILIAR

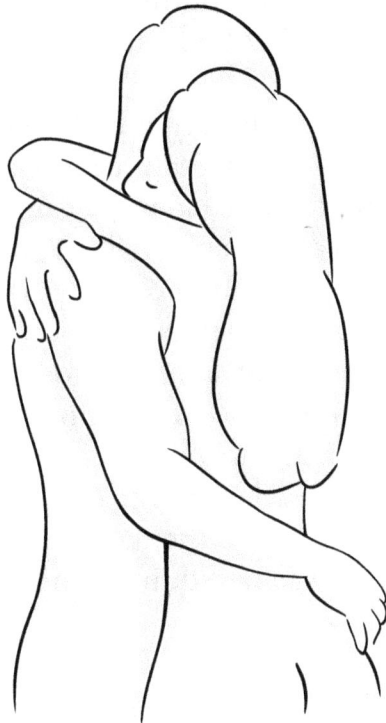

THE concept of familiar for an individual is what makes him or her feel comfortable, but that may not always be healthy in a relationship. For instance, one may have grown up in a family where his or her parents were in constant argument. In the context of *The Ultimate Intimacy Guide for Passionate People*, this is a case where sexuality may have been affected. For example, whether one is raised in an environment where sex is discussed openly and positive or in a home where sex is seen as a sin or taboo that is never to be discussed. When working with couples and doing an evaluation of one's sex history, part of the information gathered during the session has to do with past messages from childhood portrayed in the home concerning sexuality. If one party in the relationship grew up in a home where sex was not seen as negative or masturbation was not a punishable act, he or she may have a much more positive feeling about his or her body and the idea of sex and sensuality.

As we eventually meet our mate, it may not always occur to us that our parents have played an important part in shaping our ideas of sex, body image and intimacy. Negative sex parenting can result in one having sex negative ideas about oneself, and the opposite may also be true about sex positive parenting where one feels comfortable with himself or herself sexually and does not grow up with shame surrounding sex. In some instances, just looking back on how one's parents acted towards each other can be imprinted in the mind of a child as to how they are supposed to interact with others when they get older. If a child only witnesses their mom and dad being distant and not displaying any forms of affection, they may think that this is how all couples interact. If they see their mom and dad both being affectionate and loving, this will naturally be modeled to them. This is the idea of familiar—the root goes back to family or how one was raised in a family.

CASE IN POINT

This is seen in the example of a couple (Taylor and Jack) who had been married for several years and were having some issues that they came into counseling for. After going over their respective sex histories, we discovered that they were raised in diverse environments, resulting in their notion of the familiar being very different. Taylor grew up in a family where walking around naked was the norm and seeing her parents in the nude was not a big deal to her. Her parents were also very affectionate in front of her as they were constantly touching, kissing, and hugging one another. She was able to have open conversations about sex with them. On the other hand, Jack grew up in a home where his mom and dad were rarely affectionate with each other. As such, he felt very uncomfortable with his girlfriend walking around nude at home and he would even cover himself up immediately after sex. Taylor was also very touchy in public, which made him uncomfortable while Taylor found her husband to be cold and neither very affectionate nor open sexually.

This created a problem when it came to sex as he had to drink or smoke pot to let down his guard enough to feel comfortable. This also inadvertently resulted in Jack having issues performing in bed. After going over both their sex histories, I was able to conclude that both their concept of the 'familiar' was different from each other's and that expecting one another to change drastically would not resolve the problem. With a better understanding of the differences in their upbringing, we were able to explore some areas that were comfortable for both of them. This alone took a lot of work, time and acceptance from both parties, and they were eventually able to overcome this.

As couples work on the intimacy practices in the book, they will get to know their partner again on an intimate level and enjoy their time together. *The Ultimate Intimacy Guide for Passionate People* is intended to be a guidebook in which couples can write down their experiences and look back at it as a reminder of their progress or a way to refresh their knowledge of the practices while going through the course. It is a touchstone to keep on hand as a couple continually works on the ongoing process of building deeper intimacy in the partnership. Understanding the idea of familiar is an important part of the process to greater intimacy.

FOOD AND SEX HAVE A LOT IN COMMON

1. We grow up with a particular mindset about food that is passed down from our family and surroundings, just as we do with sex.
2. Each of us has an exclusive set of taste buds and enjoys different flavors and types of food, just like our unique desires towards sex.
3. Food is to be enjoyed and savored at times and at other times, we simply grab something to quell our hunger. This is the same as sex; our bodies need sex just like food. Sometimes we have to quell our sexual huger but other times, we can savor and enjoy it.
4. Food can be enjoyed alone or with others, just as the same can be done with sex.
5. The same old meal gets boring and needs spicing up at times. The same goes for our sex lives.

6. Most of us are not born chefs and are constantly learning how to whip up more interesting meals. Interesting sex needs to be learned too.

7. Spicy food can be enjoyed with a partner if they are willing to try new things with you. You can also choose to try it alone or seek out a new food buddy. This is not too different from sex. Most couples prefer to enjoy sex together but if one party is not willing, the other can either do it alone or seek out a new partner.

Instead of intercourse being the main course, it is now merely another a la carte in a satisfying sexual experience.

[TWO]

THE THREE AREAS OF TRUST

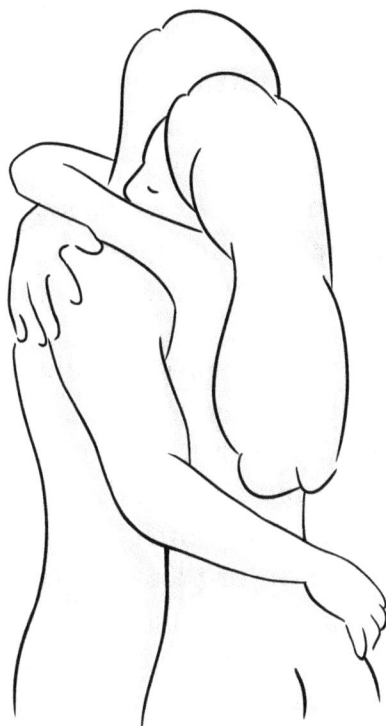

BOTH men and women need to trust their partners enough to allow themselves to be open to intimate sex. Some women are unable to reach orgasm during intercourse or have pain or fear issues regarding sex because they do not feel secure enough when they are with their partner. Trust for women can be defined by the following three levels:

1. **Physical.** Do I feel safe with my partner, knowing that he will not hurt me physically? This can also equate to a woman being physically and emotionally ready for sex. Is she aroused enough and ready? Is her partner gentle and understanding? All of these fall under physical trust.
2. **Survival.** Do we have a place to live, a roof over our heads, and enough to eat? Are the children taken care of? Can my partner protect and provide for me? While this can equate to financial stability for some, the reality is that a woman can only experience pleasurable sex and fully immerse in the sexual experience when her basic needs are met.
3. **Emotional.** Is he faithful to me? Do we have an understanding that he truly cares for me? If I get attached to him emotionally, will he be there for me when I need him? Is he going to abandon me emotionally after we have sex?

Many assume that the male population generally finds sexual intercourse enjoyable emotionally and physically as long as they are able to reach orgasm without feeling the pressure to perform. This cannot be further from the truth. A man wants to know that his partner is attracted to him, that she desires him, and is proud to be with him. In fact, his very ego has a direct impact on his performance in bed. When a man is not able to perform or please his partner, he may begin to doubt his manhood. This can then cause him to retreat emotionally and even bring about a lack of desire for sex. Others may resort to searching for fulfillment outside the relationship. As such, it is important for their partners to understand that the penis does not always have to be erect for one to be aroused and there are times when one is unable to maintain an erection even during intercourse. If this does happen, it is highly recommended to switch to another sexual activity so as to reduce the tension and help lessen anxiety. If you and your partner are giving sexual intercourse a second try after receiving help and consultation for sexual dysfunction related issues, it is even more vital to regard lovemaking as a fun and enjoyable experience and refrain from putting undue pressure on both parties.

[THREE]

Positive Sex Education

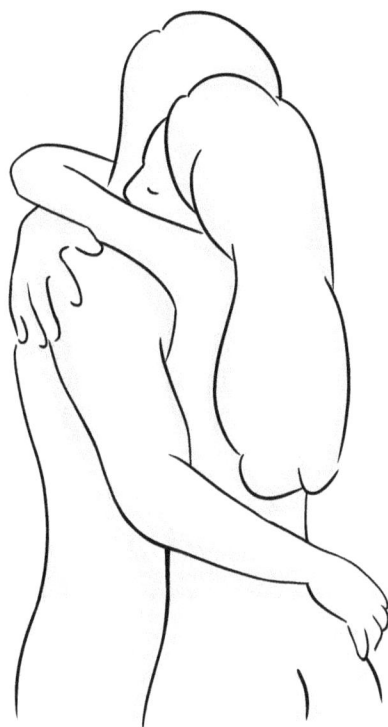

AS part of the social norm, we are not taught in school or by our parents about advanced sex education. The truth is, we are given the bare minimal amount of information and expected to somehow miraculously figure out the rest. Most of us don't even know what questions to ask our friends or where to look for solutions to our sexual problems. In recent years, there has been a growing movement towards sex positive education where professionals in the field of sexuality are speaking out about this topic. There are also more websites available than ever before where we can get help and information (a list of recommended websites is included at the end of this book).

Learning about how the female and male bodies change both sexually and mentally as one matures is extremely important. In fact, sex education plays a large role when I counsel individuals and couples. More often than not, individuals are unaware of the changes that take place in their bodies with age as well as through major life events such as parenthood, menopause, and other health related issues.

For women, going through childbirth not only changes one physically, it may also alter a couple's intimate life. Understanding that a child can have some negative effects on the intimate life is crucial. Hormones can also play a role in how a woman feels before and after childbirth, as well as throughout her life. Those who take oral contraceptives or have issues with menstruation, menopause and other health-related problems should get their hormones checked. If a woman has a hormonal imbalance, it can potentially affect her level of desire, mood and overall emotional state. In such cases, a simple test can help identify some of these issues. When counseling couples, I always recommend for a woman to have her hormones checked if she feels no sexual desire at all. A doctor can then prescribe hormone replacement if needed. There are many natural products such as hormone replacement cream and patches that are now available and these have very few negative side effects. As a hormone specialist in my own practice, I have witnessed dramatic positive results simply with the introduction of hormone replacement.

Another import factor that can affect desire and sex in general is the understanding of what it feels like to be aroused, and this is essential for a woman. The female body has erectile tissue in the vulva, clitoris and vagina that fill with blood when excited—similar to a man getting an erection. When fully aroused, the blood filled tissues become puffy and this adds much cushion in all areas of the vagina and its surrounding area. When aroused, the uterus then moves slightly, allowing the vagina to elongate and allow room for a penis to enter. Most women have at some point in their lives, experienced pain with intercourse as well as a sharp pain that may run up the lower spine or into the stomach. This can happen if the vagina is not engorged and ready for penetration. In addition, lubrication is essential. As a matter of fact, the body can produce less lubrication at some points during the menstrual cycle as well as one undergoes menopause. The same goes for the delicate tissue in the vagina and clitoris. When a woman is not fully aroused or lubricated, sex can be very much less enjoyable or even painful. As such, the act of stimulating the vulva, clitoris and vagina can also make a huge difference. For such instances, applying external lubrication that is PH-balanced will help to reduce the uncomfortable friction experienced during intercourse. However, if you or your partner are experiencing chronic dryness, it is important to seek consultation with a specialist as it may indicate a loss of estrogen or an imbalance of hormones.

Another area that many women are not fully aware of is the clitoris. While only the head is exposed, the clitoris has internal 'legs' also known as crura. The cruras wrap inside the opening of the vagina and fall in a wave-like pattern towards the cervix. In addition, every woman's vulva, clitoras and clitoral legs are unique to them.

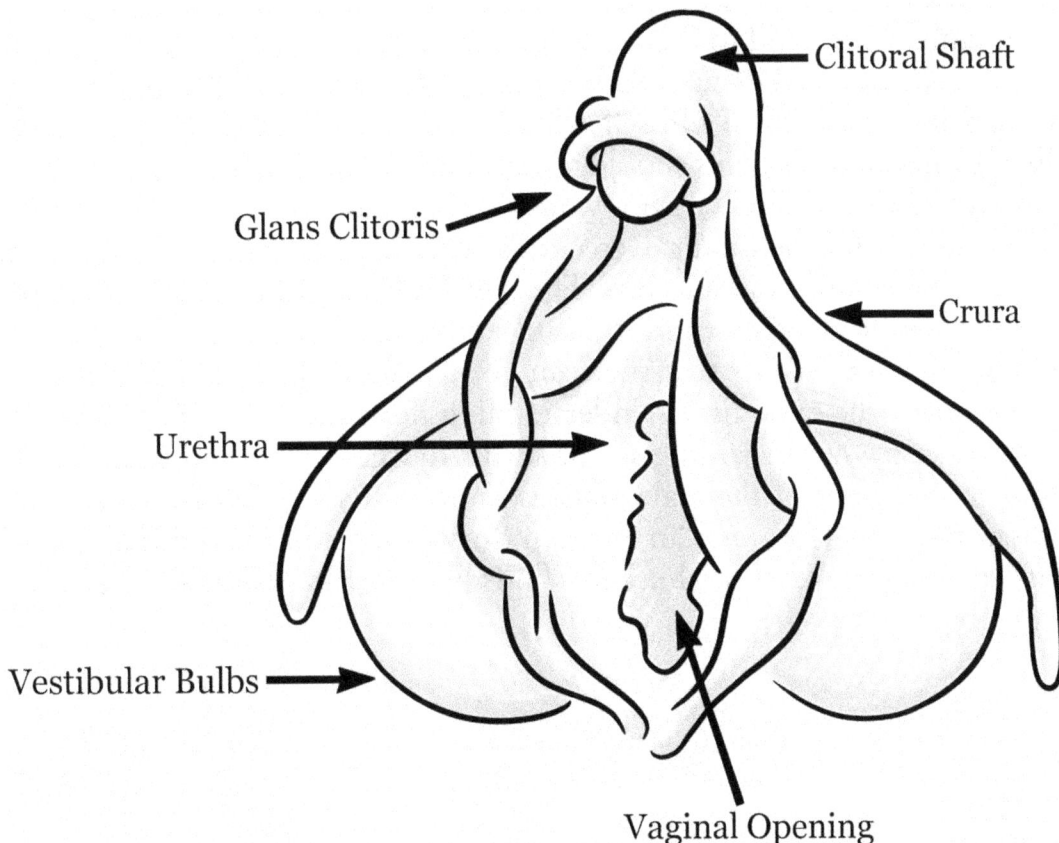

The sensitivity of the clitoral head can be likened to that of the male penis, except that it has twice as many sensitive nerve endings. Just as with the head of the penis, overstimulation of the clitoral head desensitizes and irritates the tissue and nerve endings. Using a strong vibrator or rubbing the clitoris directly can have a negative effect for some women and delay orgasm or even stop it from happening altogether. When working with couples, I explain to them that if they were to only focus on the head and not the shaft while stimulating a man's penis, it can become irritating. This is the same for the ladies. A woman's internal clitoris is like a shaft that needs to be touched as well. This can be achieved by going around the clitoral head as well as touching the g-spot. Overstimulation is usually one of the main culprits in a lack of orgasm. The other is the mental pressure to achieve orgasm. A number of women have reported a sensation of building up to an orgasm akin to climbing a mountain and just when they are about to reach the top, the orgasm subsides. When the orgasm fails to occur after the buildup, it can become extremely frustrating to a point where a woman can stop wanting to have sex or have her clitoris touched.

For men, the perception toward sex, sexual arousal, and sexual function changes as a one matures. They tend to desire more mental stimulation and direct touching of the penis—caressing, kissing and intimacy with age. In addition, the average man expects too much from himself when it comes to sexual performance. He naturally assumes that his penis should always be erect during intercourse and that losing an erection when he is with a woman is not normal. In fact, it is nothing out of the ordinary for men to have erections and then lose them during the act of intercourse at some point in their lives. The penis is in full view for men as opposed to a woman's genitals so men cannot disguise it when they lose an erection. Most men are not aware of the fact that they can be aroused with a semi-erect penis and have an orgasm at the same time. Understanding normal sexual function will help couples to address issues regarding sex or sexual dysfunctional. Educating individuals about the function of the male penis is important so that both parties do not blame themselves if a man loses an erection during intercourse, and that a woman does not needlessly feel that her husband finds her any less desirable if he does lose his erection.

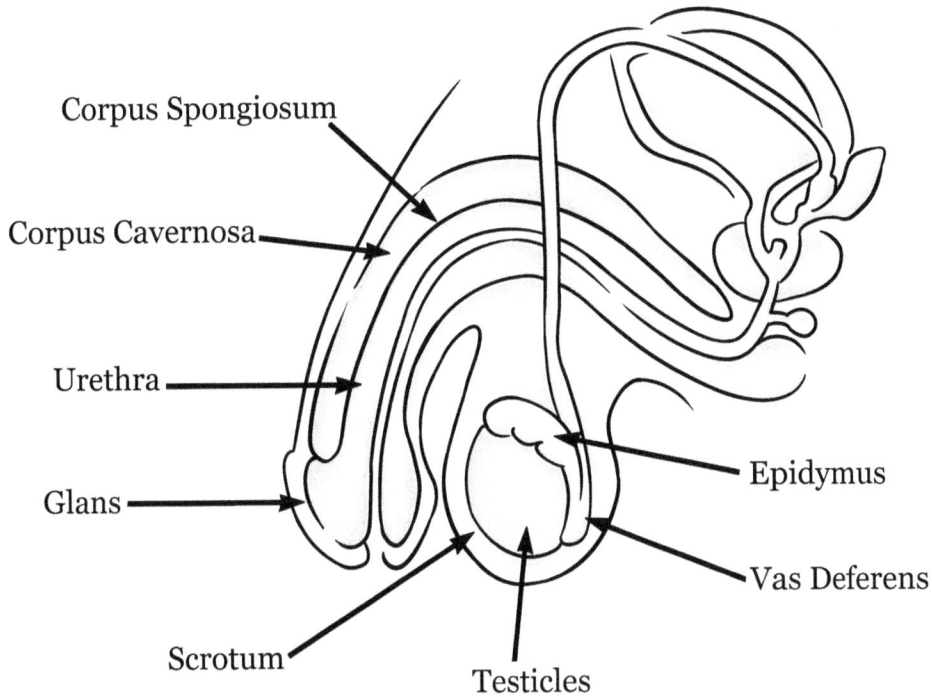

Corpus Spongiosum

Corpus Cavernosa

Urethra

Glans

Scrotum

Testicles

Epidymus

Vas Deferens

Both men and woman can have a more fulfilling sexual experience with their partner when building up the sexual desire. This brings us to the importance of both the 'Loving Exercise' on page 41 and 'Touch Exercise' on page 51. Sexual intimacy brings the mind into play as a major sex organ and for some, mental stimulation leads to better sexual intimacy and mind-blowing orgasms.

[FOUR]

UNDERSTANDING THE MIND AND BODY CONNECTION

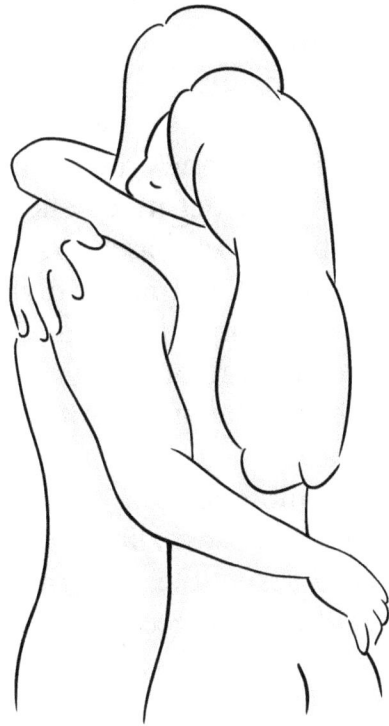

AS individuals in a relationship, we have our own notion and perception of sexual rights and responsibilities. This includes the right to sexual pleasure and the freedom of choice to take care of oneself when it comes to sexual health and pleasure. As such, I highly recommend for every one of you to give yourself the gift of pleasure through masturbation. This is the best way for one to understand how the body and mind function sexually. After all, we know our mind and body the best if given the opportunity to discover it.

Some of us may already know that while the brain is the most powerful sexual organ, it is your mind that determines how you think and feel. If your mind is focused on negative beliefs about sex, it may be difficult to experience sexual pleasure or even accept sexual pleasure from your partner. Negative beliefs about sex may cause one to pre-set limitations on the amount of pleasure that one is entitled to. These limitations can cause unhealthy sexual, emotional, mental, and even physical effects. When looking back at one's own sexual history or even childhood experiences, it may be apparent where negative beliefs about sex and pleasure may have originated. Most of these beliefs are based not in logic or nature, but rather stems from fear and control. As such, creating natural and healthy beliefs in regard to one's body and sexuality are imperative for both the enjoyment of pleasure and overall health. Learning how to reframe one's outdated belief about sexuality and self-pleasure is the best way to begin the process of change.

To move past the negative connotations of sexuality, it is important to look at some core beliefs and understand that sexuality is an integral part of who you are. You are responsible for your own sexual pleasure and you need to understand that it is healthy for your mind and body to receive pleasure. The sad truth is that the attitudes most people have regarding sex date back to the Victorian age at best.

When looking at one's own beliefs about sexual pleasure, one may ask the following basic self-reflective questions:
Do I see sexual pleasure as sacred?
Wonderful?
Sinful?
Natural?

Understanding that the answer to this question is a reflection of one's individual beliefs. This as opposed to hard and fast facts, is a positive step toward accepting that all of us have the ability to reframe our ideas surrounding sexual pleasure in a positive light.

The foundation for sexual pleasure comes from deep within you and does not involve a partner. You need to realize that the more you understand your roots, and learn to love and pleasure yourself, the greater the sexual pleasure you will then be able to enjoy. Self-knowledge comes from a conscious awareness of your own body—how to take care of it, and identifying its needs, desires and wants. In addition, taking the time to get to be well-acquainted with your body is the key to experiencing maximum sexual pleasure. This self-knowledge then translates to power with life-changing results.

Now, ask yourself the following questions:
What gives me energy?
What turns me on?
What makes me happy?

BREATHING TECHNIQUES

With regard to sexual pleasure, the correct breathing technique can be a great way to help to relax both the mind and body. While breathing is a naturally occurring event in the body, awareness and control of how you breathe can be altered. The reason is that while breathing is a part of the autonomic nervous system which is controlled by the brain stem and this part of the body is considered an involuntary action, we can override this action if we are aware of the rate, rhythm, and timing of how we breathe. This can be a powerful tool in helping with anxiety surrounding sex.

Learning how to control your breath not only helps the body to function at an optimal level, it is also vital for prolonging, increasing and maintaining sexual pleasure. Deep breathing also purifies and oxygenates the blood. Abdominal breathing, also known as diaphragmatic or pelvis breathing can also help relax the pelvic region. When we breathe, we take in oxygen and nitrogen into the lungs, hence expanding our lungs and chest cavity. This in turn, helps to oxygenate our brain and body. When we exhale on the other hand, we are releasing carbon dioxide. It is this exchange of gases as well as the techniques of inhalation and exaltation that allows the body and mind to relax. Allowing our mind to focus on breathing deeply is an effective way of taking the focus away from a potential anxious situation.

THE DEEP BREATHING EXERCISE

This exercise can be done either alone or with your partner. Begin by lying on the floor or a bed with your arms at your side and legs uncrossed. Put a small pillow under your head or neck and under your knees to make yourself more comfortable. Then close your eyes and begin breathing slowly and quietly, inhaling through your nose and exhaling through your mouth. As you breathe in and slowly feel your abdomen rise, place your hand lightly on your abdomen and concentrate on the movement of your abdomen as you inhale. Notice that your hand is being pushed upwards by your abdomen as you inhale and as you exhale, you can push down gently on the abdomen to push your breath further. Exhale twice as slowly as you inhale, making sure to exhale fully with each breath. Take your time and pause after each exhalation. With regular practice, you will notice the increase in relaxedness and energy. Once you have mastered the art of breathing, try it with your partner. This is a wonderful way to connect without words as well as to feel your partner's presence.

Practicing deep breathing while engaging in different sexual positions can create a better intimate connection. Some couples who are interested in the spiritual aspect of breath and sexuality may also want to take on some form of tantric sex. Tantra sex is an ancient Eastern spiritual practice that is believed to date back 5,000 years. Similar to yoga or the school of *zen*, it is practiced for the purpose of enlightenment and the philosophy transcends the bedroom into all aspects of life. From a tantric point of view, sex and orgasm are a symbolization of spiritual awareness at its peak. When *shiva* (as known as male energy) and *shakti* (female energy) come into a sexual union, it is believed to be the highest point of enlightenment.

> The single most important key to sex that I've yet discovered is conscious rhythmic breathing; the more you breathe the more you feel and the more you come alive. Many of us breathe only enough to survive but not to live fully. Deep breathing is a door to waking up to healing and to more personal freedom.
>
> — Annie Sprinkle, PhD., Tantrica & Ex-Porn Star

DEEP BREATHING AND SELF-PLEASURE

Breathing practices can help set the mood for self-pleasure and exploration of the body. It is important for both men and women to know their bodies and how to please themselves. Taking time to create a sacred space where you can relax. Then take control of your breathing by closing your eyes and allowing your mind to connect with your body. This is an essential to experiencing the different physical sensations of touch, tickle, pinch, pressure and pleasure. The mind body connection is extremely important when it comes to sexual intimacy because when the mind and body are not connected during sex, it becomes difficult to have an emotional connection with another person. Sex then becomes more of an act rather than a connected experience between two people. When counseling those who are experiencing disconnected sex with their partner, it has been revealed that some of the causes are attributed to past sexual trauma, body image related issues, developing an unhealthy sexual pattern over time, as well as watching sexual acts rather than experiencing sex in person over prolonged periods of time.

As you begin this self-pleasuring process, focus on touching your body while being aware of your thoughts. If you find that you are experiencing any negative thoughts, replace them with pleasant thoughts by projecting how the sensation feels good rather than what you may be doing is wrong or negative. If you find your mind drifting again, bring it back to focus with the sensation of touch. Being aware of these thoughts is the key to changing a negative thought into a pleasant feeling. When touching your body, focus on any area that may tense up and when that happens, concentrate on your breathing pattern to relax those muscles. Focus on the sensation of your skin, starting with your face, neck. Then move on to the nipples, belly, your thighs and finally, the genitals. Tease yourself if it feels good in a particular area and gradually build the tension with soft touches while slowly increasing the pressure. There are some who are unable to relax their pelvic areas alone or with a partner, and it is best recommended that they consult a somatic practitioner. Women who have experienced pelvic pain during sex, or unable to have penetration may also benefit from seeing a somatic practitioner in such instances.

During the self-pleasure exercises, it is important to refrain from not forcing yourself to do anything that is uncomfortable or painful. The idea of the experience is to associate pleasure with touch. Women who have used dilators or sex toys to try and penetrate themselves as a hasty way of seeking pleasure rather than in a self-loving way may not experience the connection of the mind and body. As such, using the finger as an initial way to explore the body is recommended. When touching the vulva, be aware of your thoughts and focus on positive feelings so as to create a new pathway. Make this experience a ritual: it can also be done in a bathtub or by applying warm soy oil. Set aside a time and space where you can create the ideal atmosphere to get yourself in the mood. Remember to take a deep breath in through your nose, filling your belly and breathe out the tension. Repeat this process several times until you feel relaxed. Allow yourself to gently seep into the process of self-pleasure as a journey, an exploration with an open mind and open heart. After all, your body is capable of feeling great pleasure and you are going to connect to that pleasure in a loving way.

If you are used to masturbating to a certain rhythm or a particular way, try introducing some variety. This can be a new way of touch, a different way of stroking or even increasing the pressure while stroking. Your experience should be one that is pleasing and therapeutic. When you have spent time exploring your body and feel comfortable with your progress, you can then share your new found pleasure with your partner.

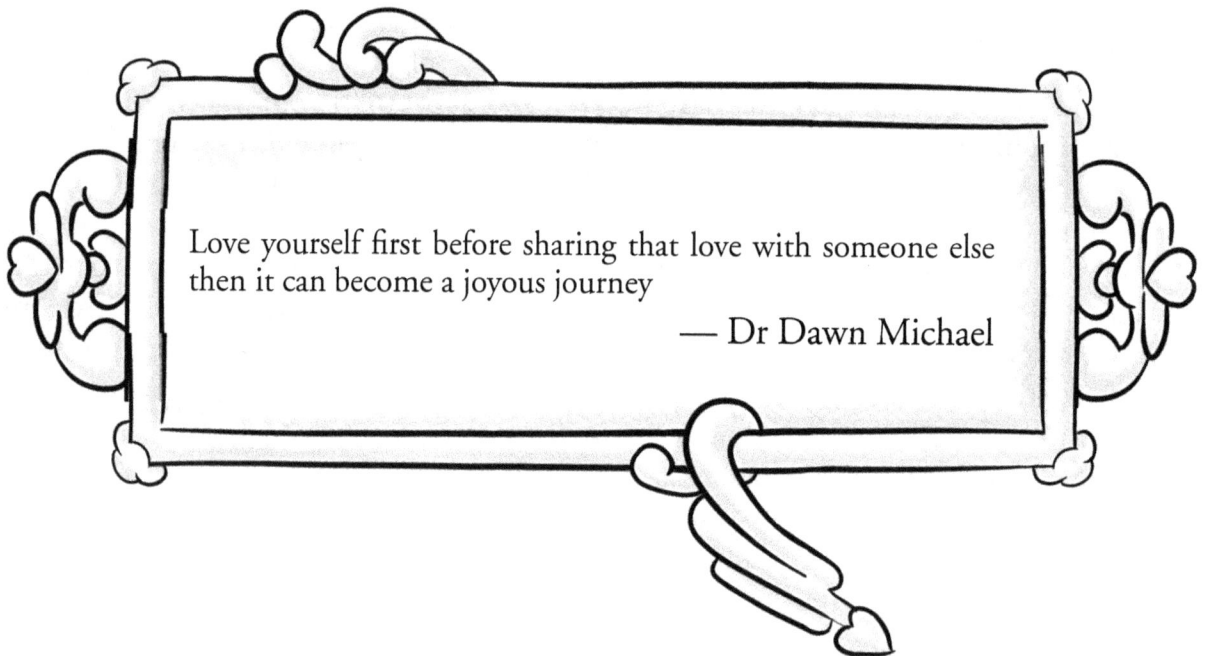

Love yourself first before sharing that love with someone else then it can become a joyous journey

— Dr Dawn Michael

[FIVE]

ART OF COMMUNICATION

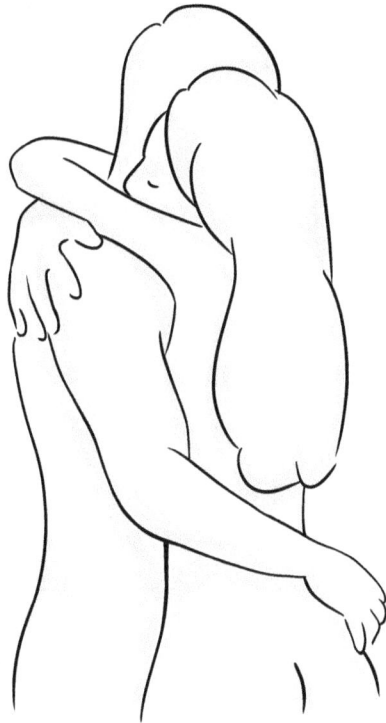

POSITIVE communication in any relationship is imperative, especially when it comes to communicating about sex. Sex is often times, a subject that people shy away from or find difficult to voice their desires. Communicating how one feels is an important aspect of a couple getting to know each other in a more intimate way. This is where the art of communication comes into play. Often times, we tell our partners **'what we don't like'** instead of **'what we do like'** and this can be taken as a form of rejection or frustration by the other party. When placed in any sexual situation where the slightest touch becomes uncomfortable, directing and showing your partner how to touch you will be better and much more appreciated rather than simply stating outright that you don't like something. That said, should you find yourself feeling uncomfortable during any part of the exercise, it is best to voice out your opinion in a positive manner.

There are instances where it is apparent that one is not aware of how a particular part of the body functions sexually and this boils down to the lack of knowledge of one's body on a more intimate level. One of the goals of the intimacy exercises is for one to rediscover his or her body in order to demonstrate to one's partner what feels good to them. This can also be achieved through masturbation, be it solo or in front of a partner as more often than not, one can be out of touch with his or her own body. This will be discussed further in the chapter on masturbation and body exploration.

Words and ideas can be expressed verbally or non-verbally and knowing how to communicate is equally important. The act of touching is a wonderful way to communicate non-verbally and in some cases can even resolve an issue much more quickly than simply bantering on about a problem endlessly. Before an argument gets potentially heated, try giving a simple hug or kiss to defuse the situation—you will see the results! When it comes to pleasure trying to explain to your partner what feels good sexually, it may be a better idea to take their hands and simply show them what feels good to you or by doing it to them instead. Non-verbal forms of communication such as a hug or a kiss can communicate love or intimacy in a way that extends beyond words

Knowing when to communicate with your partner is especially important if you want them to hear what you have to say. Timing in this instance can literally make or break an argument. Forcing your partner to respond when he or she is not ready or pushing your own agenda upon him or her can aggravate the situation. Always remember that what you feel about a situation is your opinion and it may differ from your partner's. Be respectful and give your partner the option to speak when he or she is ready instead of jumping on him or her in a bid to get your point across. Asking someone to change or to adopt your opinion is not an easy task—just think about how difficult it is for you to accept a new pattern or idea at times.

This brings us back to 'The Concept of the Familiar' (page 5) in which what may seem familiar and absolutely correct to you may not be the same for your partner. As such, helping your partner to understand why you feel strongly about a certain idea or opinion is the best way to help in improving the situation. This is illustrated in one of my counseling sessions where a couple (Helen and Fred) who sought my advice.

CASE IN POINT

Fred mentioned that he and Helen were rarely having sex and she always seemed angry with him. Upon further probing, Helen stated that she felt that Fred never listens to her. She also added that they had too many unresolved issues and that he never wanted to face them together with her and even went as far as to avoid talking about the problems altogether. Over time, she began to feel resentful and was no longer attracted to him. Helen added that she would choose to bring up the issues that were upsetting her during car rides as she had assumed that this would be a good opportunity to get Fred's full attention. However, he would either get upset with her or simply tuned her out. Whereas from Fred's point of view, all he wanted was to get his wife safely to her destination. It turned out that what she thought was an excellent opportunity to iron out their differences became a source of distraction that got him upset, and eventually made matters worse. When I asked Fred if he felt that it was not important to hear what his wife's concerns were, he explained that he did care but felt attacked most of the time and would rather choose to tune her out instead. I then asked Fred if he would prefer his wife to allow him the option of choosing when they could speak about their issues so that so he would be better able to listen to her. He agreed to my suggestions and that was just the first step to mending their relationship. We then focused on how Helen presented her problems and voiced her unhappiness.

This is where the art of communication comes into play. If you want to get your point across to your partner effectively, you need to choose the appropriate time. In addition, refrain from accusing or putting your partner down as this will only make them feel like they have to defend themselves. When expressing one's feelings, it is also recommended to use the 'I' statements as much as possible. An excellent example of this is that of another couple, Linda and Eric, that I counseled.

CASE IN POINT

Linda was upset that Eric never lifted a finger to help her clean the dishes after dinner and he explained that he stopped volunteering to do so because he did not know exactly what she wanted him to do and that he could never get it right anyway. With some guidance, Linda began to communicate her thoughts and requests in a clearer manner. By simply rephrasing herself to 'I feel frustrated when I ask for your help in the kitchen and you don't do what I ask.' instead of 'You never help me in the kitchen when I ask you.', Eric was able to see the source of her unhappiness. In addition, adding specific descriptions such as 'When I ask you to help me in the kitchen, it will be great if you could put the dishes in the dishwasher, please.' instead of 'Please clean the dishes up and leaving them out to dry out.' played a huge part in helping Linda to get her message across effectively. Now, imagine this very scenario happening in the bedroom and how often we do not tell our partners exactly about our preferences as well as fail to explain to our partners what to do to please us sexually.

When couples have been together for an extended period of time, they tend to get complacent and take the fact that their bodies and minds age over time for granted. Hence, focusing on their present selves and current state of mind becomes one of the objectives of the intimacy exercises in this guidebook as couples explore new unchartered territories with an open mind and open heart. There are individuals who do get caught up in the past from time to time, as they find themselves being unable to move forward. In such instances, they may find it important to set up a counseling session so as to find out whether there might be a deeper problem that needs to be dealt with first. Overall, couples will greatly benefit from working as a team at resolving the issues.

In some rare cases, one may also come to the realization that he or she no longer wants to be in a relationship, or that there may be past sexual trauma that has resurfaced that needs to be sorted out first. Nonetheless, it is important to remember that this is a new chapter in one's life and that it will be difficult to fully benefit from this process if past grievances are continuously being brought up. While it is important to confront the history of past negative experiences it helps the couple to move forward together, there are instances where reliving the past or eliciting negativity will only impede the process of learning to be more intimate. This brings us the next chapter on masturbation and body exploration.

[SIX]

REFRAMING AN IDEA

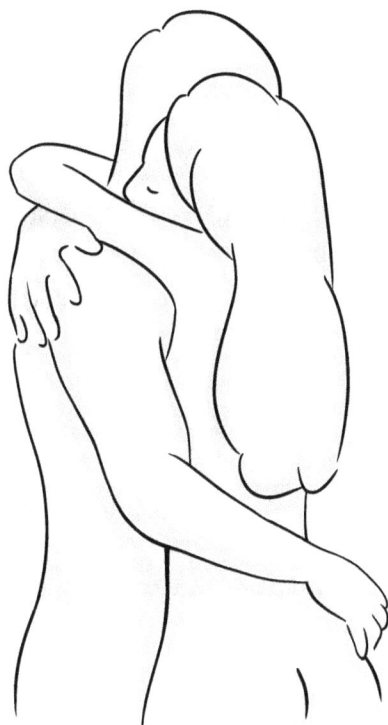

WHEN one has a preconceived notion about how something needs to be, this becomes a familiar idea. Often times, this may not always be best for a relationship. By understanding that an idea can be interpreted in a different way or a new perspective, we can reframe our opinions and thoughts. The technique of reframing is especially important when couples are faced with issues related to sex. There are some individuals who have misconceptions about sex and sexuality in terms of what is acceptable. The theory of reframing comes into the picture here. When we attempt to reframe a problem or sculpt a new solution based on a different understanding, this becomes a useful tool in coping with one's past sexual experiences, or how one may have been brought up to think about sex in terms of childhood experiences, religious views and societal normative.

An individual may have the idea that he or she could never perform or be comfortable performing a certain sexual act or position. However, if he or she now regards it from a different perspective that is based on sex positive education, his or her mindset are then shifted or reframed. For instance, there are some who may have been told at an early age that sex is a dirty act and they should feel ashamed when they are masturbating or having sex with a partner. This may very well further justify their sense of guilt by solely having sex in the missionary position because it is the only position they find tolerable. Helping these individuals to reframe this ingrained idea and to understand that there is more than one way to look at a situation can help to change their belief that experimenting with sex in other positions is unacceptable and perverse. Bryan and Samantha a couple that counseled previously, were only able to have sex in the missionary position and with the lights off because Samantha was taught that it was the only acceptable position to have sex. By reframing her idea of sexual position as well as introducing her to other new ideas, we were able to encourage her to try some different positions featured in 'The Intimacy Exercises'.

Couples who have issues concerning oral sex can also benefit from reframing one's mindset. When one begins to view oral sex as an enjoyable act as opposed to a duty or something dirty, this can have a dramatic change in a couple's sex life. In fact, sex education surrounding oral sex is essential in order for one to not only understand how to please one's partner, but also to help drive away any misconceptions he or she may have about oral sex. Giving pleasure to one's partner orally and watching his or her reaction in return can alter the dynamic of this interaction. This is simply achieved by reframing one's mindset. The same goes for masturbation.

One's negative views regarding masturbation or the idea of touching oneself for pleasure needs to be reframed in order for one to fully understand your body on an intimate level.

The key is changing one's perception. In addition, adding a dash of laughter and levity to this series of intimacy exercises in this guidebook can help a couple relax and make them realize how silly some of their preconceived notions may have been. The more you and your partner can laugh together, the easier it will be for both of you to understand and embrace the idea that sex is meant to be fun and enjoyable! As you go through this guidebook, you will now have the opportunity to learn more about yourself and open your mind to new possibilities surrounding sexuality and intimacy.

Trying something new helps to open up amazing possibilities of seeing the same subject in a different light.

— Dr. Dawn Michael

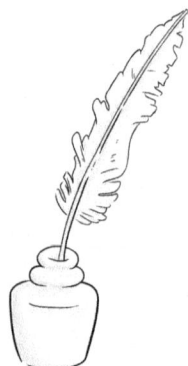

NOTES

Use the subsequent pages to come up with some misconceptions you may have about sex, your body image or sexuality. Then reframe these in a positive light. An example is 'I don't want my husband to see me naked because I am embarrassed.' instead of 'My husband gets turned on when he sees me naked and I am denying him that pleasure.'

Keep adding positive reasons to the list as you go through 'The Intimacy Exercises'. You can do this alone or with your partner. As you move on to the later exercises in this guidebook, you may want to refer to this page and add more notes.

_____

_____

_____

_____

_____

_____

_____

NOTES

NOTES

_____

_____

_____

_____

_____

_____

_____

_____

_____

_____

NOTES

_____

_____

_____

_____

_____

_____

_____

_____

_____

_____

NOTES

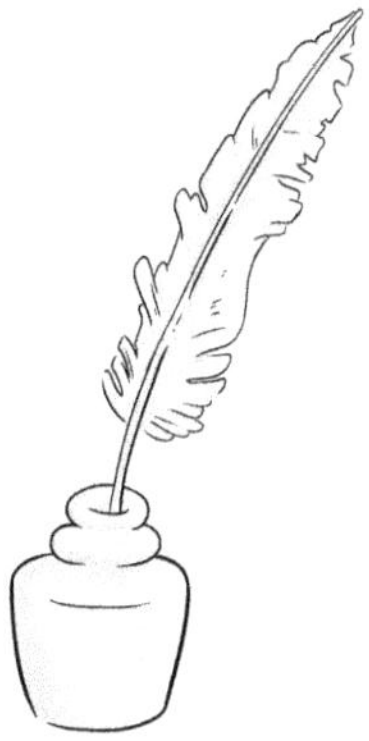

NOTES

_____

_____

_____

_____

_____

_____

_____

_____

_____

NOTES

_____

_____

_____

_____

_____

_____

_____

_____

_____

_____

[SEVEN]

SETTING THE GROUNDWORK

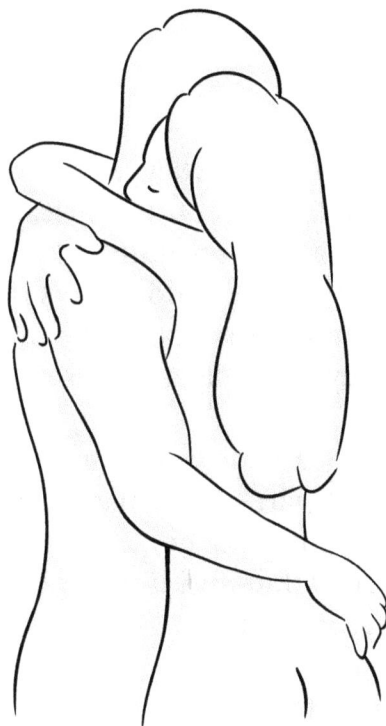

BEFORE starting 'The Intimacy Exercises', it is important to set the proper groundwork. The six golden rules in this chapter will put in place some safety measures and boundaries so that you and your partner can enjoy the intimacy exercises at your own pace while reaping its full benefits. This chapter also covers the concept of intimate space and how you and your partner can create an ideal environment.

You may want to purchase a few of these items beforehand to enhance the experience:

1. Blindfold
2. Candles
3. Soft pillow
4. Water based lubrication

The first rule is that you and your partner are responsible for taking turns to initiate each intimacy exercise. The person initiating leads the exercise throughout the session. When a couple shares the responsibility of initiating an exercise, this takes pressure off the other, along with the rejection that so often ensues. Alternating also gives the party who is usually more passive the responsibility of claiming his or her preferred expression of intimacy. Flipping a coin is a great way to decide who starts!

Secondly, both of you need to swap roles and revisit the same exercise in the same week. This is an essential part of intimacy counseling and will be an integral part of all the exercises in this guidebook. For many couples, initiating sex or lovemaking is often a one-sided affair and it is now time to break this pattern that can often become deeply entrenched in long-term relationships.

The third rule is with regard to preparing an intimate space. This will then be your safe and inviting space for what is to follow. The initiator of a particular session will be the one responsible for making sure that the space (bedroom or room) is comfortable. This includes cleaning and decluttering the space, and adjusting the lighting and temperature to help set the perfect mise-en-scène. Many couples forget that having a space of their own to make love in is important as it allows them to reconnect and take their minds off external stress factors. An intimate space is one that is free from the reminders of work, children, or anything other than comfort. As you and your partner go through the practices, you may find yourselves wanting to improve the intimate space further by adding new bedding, a coat of paint to the walls, and dimmer lighting. Couples are also encouraged to look at pictures of bedrooms together and decide on how their dream bedroom will look—one that should provide the option of accommodating soft sounds, dim lighting, and tranquility. Having a new touch to existing furnishing can provide a refreshing environment to experiment with a new sexual position.

Fourthly, you and your partner are highly encouraged to work on each exercise for at least 20 minutes. That said, both of you are completely free from the pressure to perform. If one of you is aroused at the end of the session, you are encouraged to take care of your own sexual needs, without expecting your partner to join in.

Next, it is highly recommended for you and your partner to write down your feelings in the respective 'Notes' section in this guidebook and share these with each other. Whenever possible, it is best that both of you also spend to have a discussion about your experiences or to share your ideas in a positive light after each session. However, bear in mind that this is strictly an avenue to encourage positive feedback and not to pressure each other to speak.

Last but not least, follow the order of exercises listed in this guidebook as much as possible. These exercises have been specially developed to facilitate a couple's journey of introducing intimacy in a relationship. It also establishes the initiating process so that both of you can immerse yourselves progressively.

Now that we've set the groundwork, let's proceed to have some real fun!

[EIGHT]

THE LOVING EXERCISE

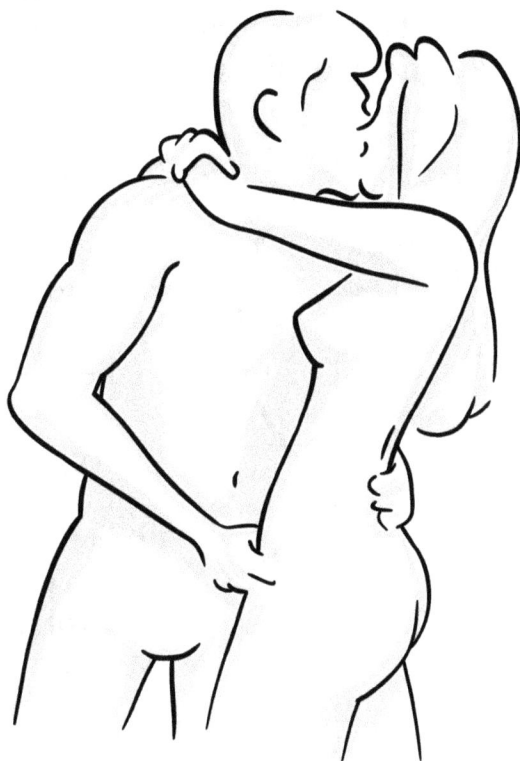

'THE LOVING EXERCISE' is based on the concept of how a person wants 'to feel loved' by his or her partner. When working with couples during counseling sessions, I usually ask each individual to write down five things that make them feel loved by their partner and to include specific examples. This exercise has proved to be very effective when done in an honest and positive manner. The end result is a couple getting to know each other better through the process.

In this exercise, both you and your partner need to write down and clearly define five ways that make you feel loved. Then take turns reading it out loud to your partner. This is the time to give your partner your utmost undivided attention. One of the objectives in this exercise is to cultivate the practices of active listening and communication with an open mind. Then take turns to clarify your doubts if necessary. This is essentially a follow-up on chapter five's 'Reframing Exercise'.

I feel loved when my partner makes me feel safe. I feel safe when my partner shares what he is thinking with me instead of having me to guess his thoughts.

I feel loved when my partner shows me that she loves me by being physically affectionate. I would like her to kiss me each morning and show her feelings through physical acts such as hugging me.

Here are some examples of what other couples have discussed during the exercises. These preferences often relate back to childhood experiences of what the concept of love felt to them.

Keep in mind that the concept of 'feeling loved' spells differently to everyone. It can mean a particular action, words, form of physical affection, or even sex. The important thing to note during this exercise is that this it is not about your partner, but you! Couples can quite often live together for years and never come to understand why their partner is not reciprocating their displays of love and affection. This is simply because we all have different ways of expressing and demonstrating how we like to be loved.

Case in point

An excellent example is a couple that I counseled Bruce and Pattie. Bruce and Pattie were both in their early 50s and were rediscovering their relationship after they had sent their last kid off to college. They had been married for 24 years and felt that they had lost touch with each other as well as the spark in the bedroom. Bruce had always initiated sex in the marriage but over the last five years, he stopped doing so. As such, their sex lives had dwindled drastically. During the counseling session, Bruce and Pattie were asked to write down what made them feel loved. Bruce indicated that he felt loved when his wife desired him. Pattie was surprised by what Bruce had written because she felt that over the years, he was not that interested in sex with her. He also added that she could have showed that she still desired him if she had initiated sex instead. On the other hand, Pattie had always assumed that men needed to be the ones in charge of initiating sex and thought Bruce simply did not wish to be intimate with her if he did not ask for it.

> I feel loved when my partner makes me dinner.

> I feel loved when we have sex. I would like my partner to take the time to kiss me or rub my back before and after sex.

A huge part of the process of the exercise was then focused on working out what Pattie could do in order to demonstrate to Bruce that she desired him. With this information, we were able to work through the intimacy exercises and have both Pattie and Bruce take on equal responsibility in initiating sex.

Some of you may realize that the most interesting part about this exercise is that no matter how long a couple has been together, they will always be learning something new about each other at the end of the session. This is because as evolving individuals, we have very specific needs and desires at different points in our lives.

When doing this exercise, write down five sentences and then break them down into standalone actions. Use the following writing pages in this guide to serve as a handy reference for your relationship.

NOTES

_____

_____

_____

_____

_____

_____

_____

_____

_____

_____

NOTES

NOTES

_____

_____

_____

_____

_____

_____

_____

_____

_____

_____

NOTES

NOTES

_____

_____

_____

_____

_____

_____

_____

_____

_____

_____

Notes

_____

_____

_____

_____

_____

_____

_____

_____

_____

_____

[NINE]

THE TOUCH EXERCISE

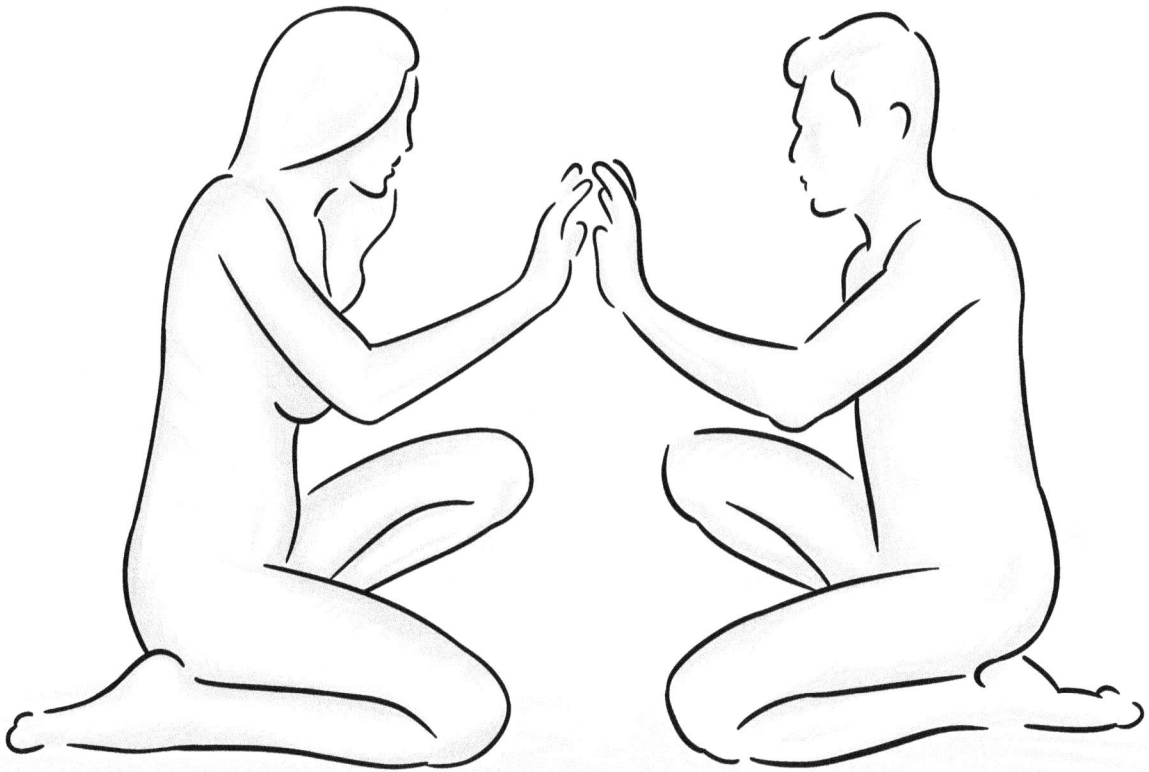

DO you know how your partner likes to be touched? The act of touching is a wonderful way to connect with your partner and communicate your emotions in a non-verbal manner. Remember the times when you both spent hours bickering over a small issue and how a simple hug was the solution? 'The Touch Exercise' is a powerful yet simple exercise to warm you up before moving into 'The Intimacy Exercises'.

Begin the Touch Exercise by taking turns to touch each other's arm: turn the arm around with your palms facing up and gently touch your partner's arm. When doing this exercise, look into your partner's eyes from time to time. Maintaining eye contact while touching each other, it can be both sensually powerful and soothing at the same time. Take this opportunity to show your partner how you like to be touched. More often than not, we touch each other in a petting manner. In this exercise, the key is to try and experiment with different sensual energies and alternative types of physical contacts. Then ask your partner what feels best.

When asking couples to do this particular exercise in my office, I will usually have one person seated and the other standing. The latter is than asked to go behind the former and to touch his or her head and face. I have observed that some males have said that they did not like having their face touched because it resembled more of one petting a dog or soothing a child. In short, there was no sensuality to it. When I redirected the ladies to touch their partners with more passion and with increased pressure, the general feedback as that this was much more preferable. The contrary was for the men who were more often than not, too rough and rushed when touching their female partners. This is because women have a lot more nerve receptors and hence, they tend to have a much more delicate and sensitive skin. Men should pay attention to such details and make an effort to be gentler when touching their partners in this exercise. On the other hand, a man may prefer a stronger touch. Using one's lips and tongue as well as other parts of the body while touching can also introduce new sensations that go beyond just using hands.

For this first exercise, simply start with the arm. This is an area that is safe for most people and a neutral place to start. One can then continue with the head and face and proceed down from there. When touching the arm, start with the shoulder and apply a single long stroke from the tip of the middle finger. Begin with this slow sensual touch without breaking the stroke from start to finish. The individual receiving this first touch can close his or her eyes and focus on the sensation. Start at the top of the shoulder and move your hands in one long stroke down to the tip of your fingers to evoke a feeling of completion. Women tend to prefer being touch top-down from the side of the body and from the upper inner thigh down to the side of the foot, finishing at the toe. On the other hand, men prefer to have themselves lying face up in the bed with their partners rubbing from under the armpit all the way down the side to the toes with both hands whilst standing over them. Try different parts of the body with your partner and then talk about what feels good for both of you. There are a wide variety of touch—sensual touch, loving touching, playful touching, healing touch, rough touching, teasing touching, just to name a few. The objective here is to experiment and have a feel of the different types of touch.

After touching each other's arm, spend the next 20 minutes touching and exploring your partner's hair, face, neck, hands and arms in the very way you would like to be touched. Then have them do the same to you. A simple touch is a very powerful thing and can very often evoke emotions and sensations that cannot be captured by words. The act of touching can activate a deep sense of connection and an immediate understanding of what your partner desires. At the same time, touching can also release powerful emotions that may have been buried in the past. As with the other exercises, always be aware of how your touch is affecting your partner. Always make a conscious effort to talk about and be respectful of your partner's feelings.

CASE IN POINT

An excellent example is another couple that I have counseled. Erika and Jeremy have been married for over 20 years and Erika had subconsciously held onto the pain of a miscarriage and I had asked the couple to do 'The Touch Exercise' at home. Jeremy was gently touching her stomach and hips when she began to cry as she felt pain in her pelvis and lower abdomen. Sensing her distress, he then stopped and gave her a hug and held her as she let go of her emotional pain. It then began to dawn upon Erika that she had been holding on to the pain of the miscarriage that happened so many years ago. It was a subject that the couple had avoided speaking about and Erika did not realize that she was holding on to the emotional pain in her pelvic area. During the couple's follow-up session, it became apparent that we needed to look into helping Erika fully let go of her grieve before we could move forward with the other exercises.

Erika and Jeremy's case shows the important of touch and how it can affect us on more than just the physical level. Now, it is your turn to try out this exercise with your partner, jot down both your thoughts in the following 'Notes' section and revisit your experiences later. Upon completion of 'The Touch Exercise', you are now ready to move on to the set of intimacy exercises in the next chapter.

NOTES

_____

_____

_____

_____

_____

_____

_____

_____

_____

NOTES

_____

_____

_____

_____

_____

_____

_____

_____

_____

_____

NOTES

NOTES

_____

_____

_____

_____

_____

_____

_____

_____

_____

_____

NOTES

NOTES

_____

_____

_____

_____

_____

_____

_____

_____

_____

_____

[TEN]

THE INTIMACY PRACTICES

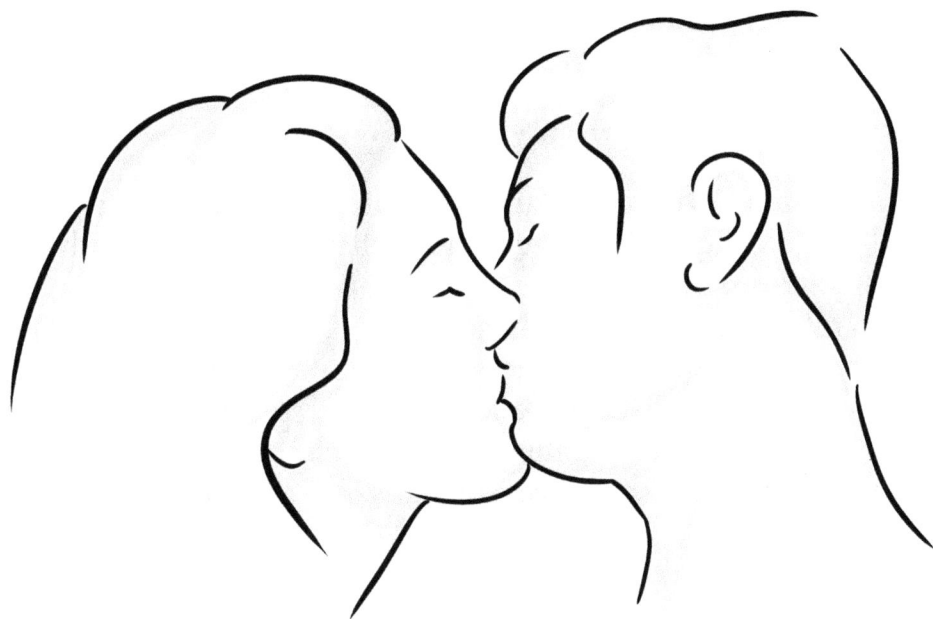

AFTER completing the series of exercises in the earlier chapters, it is now the time to move onto 'The Intimacy Practices'. These practices are to be done in the nude with you and your partner taking turns to finish practices 1 (page 64) and 2 (page 72) on the same day. The remaining practices can be done on separate days. After each practice, write down how you feel and sensations, emotions, or any discomfort you might have experienced. The idea of an intimate touch is very different from the act of simply having sex as the former can trigger deep feelings and past emotions. The following series of intimacy practices are designed to bring you and your partner closer together on both an emotional and physical level through pure enjoyment and pleasure. If you are not yet comfortable doing these in the nude, this needs to be one of your goals. When doing the intimacy practices, there are many ways to touch your partner: using your fingers, mouth, body and even the tongue. Experiencing different forms of touch not only feel pleasurable, it also adds variety and excitement.

HANDS EXERCISE

Intimacy practice 1 starts with the 'Hands Exercise'. The purpose of this warm-up exercise is to allow you and your partner to feel what it is like to be submissive and to take control. This also creates a connection between the two of you before any progression into full body touching. You and your partner are encouraged to come up with different terms such as the leader and the follower, or the explorer and the subject. This is always an interesting exercise for me to witness as some couples are perfectly fine following and leading and others clearly have problems allowing the other person to lead or initiate. Eye contact is also another part of the exercise. Looking each other in the eye for an extended time can be connecting for some people and difficult for others.

CASE IN POINT

Tim and Nancy, needed my help in getting them past an infidelity issue. Tim had recently ended the affair and both of them decided to give their marriage another shot. Nancy agreed and they contacted me for help. We talked about what lead up to the affair and how it happened. They then revealed that intimacy has always been a problem throughout the marriage. While Tim wanted more intimacy, Nancy had been unable to do so. She was aware that the affair was a result of this and now wanted to deal with the root of the problem—which was her disinterest in sex. After a few counseling sessions, I decided that the couple was now ready to get started on 'The Intimacy Practices'. However, I wanted them to go through the 'Hands Exercise' in my office first to see if there may be any other potential issues that may surface. When asked to hold each other's gaze while doing the exercise, Nancy began to tear up and started to cry. Upon seeing the pain in his wife's eyes, Tim also began to tear up as they held each other's gaze. No words were exchanged throughout this period and there was simply no need for them to. Tim then put his arms around Nancy as she allowed him to hold her. When they both released their holds on each other, it seemed as though a weight had been lifted from Nancy's shoulders. They then repeated this exercise again from start to completion. This was the beginning of the healing process for Tim and Nancy.

To begin the 'Hands Exercise', stand approximate one foot part from your partner and look into each other's eyes. Then place your hands together upright, facing out and touch each other palm to palm.

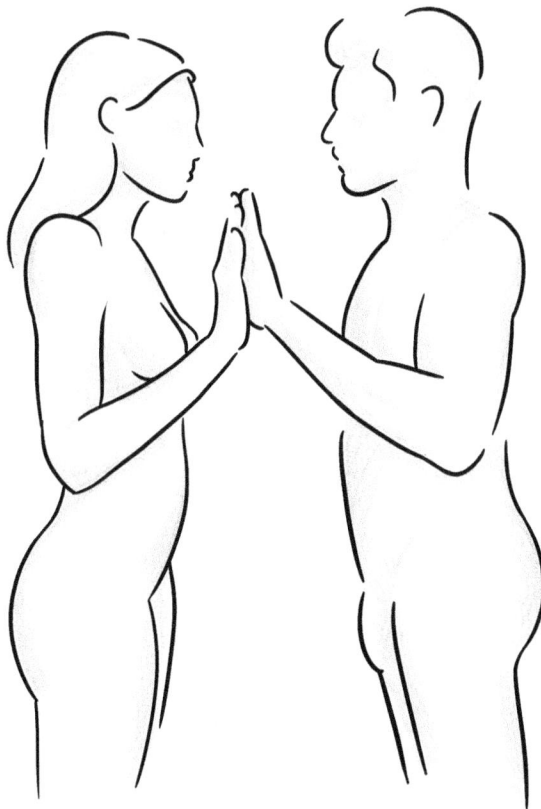

Next, move your palms in small circular directions and alternate this between pushing forward, up and down and to the side, with your partner following. This helps to set the tone for the rest of the exercise and can be done nude or dressed. Do this for about five minutes and take turns leading. Then take turns and repeat this exercise with your eyes closed. Finish this exercise by opening your eyes and giving each other a hug and kiss to create a more connecting experience. For some couples, this exercise can be difficult. As such, always spend some time talking about the exercise at the end of each session. I have observed that a couple usually has a difficult time looking into each other's eyes in instances where the trust had been broken or when there is a lack of respect in the relationship. If you find that it is difficult to look your partner in the eye, then there are some deeper issues that the two of you will need to address or see a counselor to have them resolved before proceeding with the other practices in this book.

INTIMACY PRACTICE 1

If both you and your partner had your clothes on while doing the 'Hands Exercise', now is the time to take them off and touch each other's bodies with your hands, lips or even rubbing your body against theirs. The easiest way to do this practice is for both of you to be on the bed with the follower lying face down and the leader at the side. The leader then starts with the top of the head and works his or her down to the toes. This can be done with the hands, body or mouth. The objective here is to take the time and feel the sensations of the skin, the change in energy level and to reap the benefits of this practice. When doing this practice, focus on how you feel rather than what your partner is thinking. This is not a simple massage but more of an exploration of your partner's body as well as how your body feels against theirs. While exploring, pay attention to the way the skin feels, the reaction to a certain touch, and the exchange of energy. Repeat this practice with your eyes closed and then take turns. If you find your mind drifting off during this 20-minute exercise, pull your focus back to a part of your partner's body that pleases you or the feel of his or her skin or reaction to your touch. Try to stay connected to your partner for the entire practice as much as possible. Some couples have reported when that when they were the followers, they could feel when their partner was mentally present or when they were drifting off.

After completing the practice, spend some time talk about how both of you felt during the session, the sensations experienced and what you have both learned.

The purpose of the all the practices in this guidebook is to enable you and your partner to connect with each other without the pressure to perform. As such, if you feel that your partner is losing focus or connection, bring it up gently and talk about it. This may be something that they are unaware of and could be the key in creating a stronger physical and emotional connection.

NOTES

_____

_____

_____

_____

_____

_____

_____

_____

_____

_____

NOTES

_____

_____

_____

_____

_____

_____

_____

_____

_____

NOTES

NOTES

_____

_____

_____

_____

_____

_____

_____

_____

_____

NOTES

_____

_____

_____

_____

_____

_____

_____

_____

_____

_____

NOTES

_____

_____

_____

_____

_____

_____

_____

_____

_____

INTIMACY PRACTICE 2

KISSING EXERCISE

'Intimacy Practice 2' starts with the 'Kissing Exercise'. Kissing is an integral part of intimacy and it is highly encouraged for this to be incorporated into the rest of the intimacy practices in this guidebook. The goal of this exercise is for both you and your partner to show how one likes to be kissed. This is also a fun way to experiment with various ways of kissing with your partner—soft tender kissing, tongue kissing, deep passionate kissing, or exploratory kissing. It can literally be a mouth-opening experience for some couples!

In fact, our lips are actually much more sensual than we think. One of the most sensitive parts of the body is under the front lip. Try taking the tip of your tongue and rubbing it under the top of your lip, and you will feel the tissue connecting your gums and lip. Doing this to your partner is similar to simulating oral sex and can be very arousing. Kissing is one way to get aroused, especially for women, because small amounts of testosterone are released from the man's saliva into the woman's mouth. This is believed to not just activate the feelings of arousal but also serve to enhance the sexual connection. As such, kissing is a great way to tease your partner as well as to slowly get him or her into the mood. When couples kiss without the expectation of it leading to anything else, a simple make out session can invoke feelings of desire. Have fun taking turns and learn something new about each other.

This practice is similar to 'Intimacy Practice 1' except that your partner will now need to lie facing upwards instead of lying on their stomach. Explore your partner's face, lips, hair and ears using your fingers as well as your mouth. Have your partner close his or her eyes while laying down. They can also choose to put on a blindfold on if desired. Then work your way down the body, including the neck, the chest, stomach but avoiding the genitalia area. Use your hands to gently rub the side of your partner, starting from the armpit down to the feet with long gentle strokes. Spread your partner's legs and run your hands from the upper thigh down to the feet, avoiding the genital areas. You can also use your mouth as well and run kisses along your partner's body or rub your body against theirs. Then take turns and repeat this practice. Observe your partner's reactions throughout this session. The objective is not to have sexual intercourse but to explore the many ways touch can increase and deepen intimacy. It is highly recommended for couples to refrain from touching the genitalia area so as to prevent arousal and instead, draw focus to the more subtle experiences and sensations that can lead to deeper connection through this practice. Progressively, couples who are more experienced and comfortable doing such practices in the nude after completing the entire series of intimacy practices can use these as a foreplay to intercourse. Do note that if either of you does get aroused, that is not the intention of the practice, nor is it the responsibility of the other to pleasure the former. As with all earlier practices, always remember that open communication is key to reaping the full benefits of these sessions.

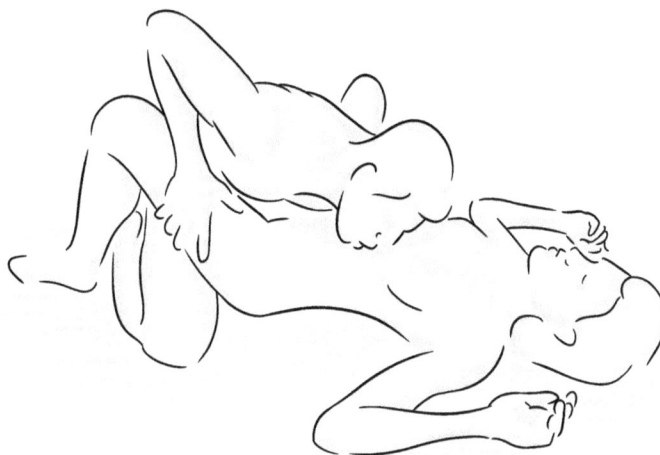

STAYING CONNECTED

One of the main objectives of the intimacy practices is to explore the themes of sexuality, intimacy, connecting, and healing. For some, the act of intercourse can cause anxiety and there are others who may mentally and emotionally disconnect themselves while having sex. This is also known as mentally checking out. Individuals who have had past sexual trauma or performance anxiety may take to mentally checking out during sex. In these cases, sex may then be experienced as a function rather than a connection with one's partner. An individual who is fearful of connecting on an emotional level may resort to intercourse as a way of avoiding confronting his or her deeper feelings. For some, the act of intercourse can even be compared to washing dishes and provides the opportunity for the mind to drift away. When this happens, a couple cannot experience true sexual intimacy. With the help of the exercises in this guidebook, couples can learn how to keep themselves mentally engaged in the moment of lovemaking and establish a mind and body connection. However, the act of intercourse will only be introduced at the last stage as it can disrupt the process of reconnecting one's mind with one's body.

NOTES

_____

_____

_____

_____

_____

_____

_____

_____

_____

_____

_____

NOTES

_____

_____

_____

_____

_____

_____

_____

_____

_____

_____

NOTES

_____

_____

_____

_____

_____

_____

_____

_____

_____

NOTES

_____

_____

_____

_____

_____

_____

_____

_____

_____

_____

NOTES

_____

_____

_____

_____

_____

_____

_____

_____

_____

NOTES

_____

_____

_____

_____

_____

_____

_____

_____

_____

_____

INTIMACY PRACTICE 3

Having explored the more subtle dynamics of touch in the previous practice, this intimacy practice is about genital play and the different pleasure zones for men and women. Relaxation is the crux of this intimacy practice. Begin the practice by doing the 'The Deep Breathing Exercise' on page 19 with your partner.

The exercise should be done with you and partner naked. Begin this intimacy practice with either of you laying on the bed and the other positioned close. You also have the option of using a chair to explore the body, the follower sits in the chair and the leader is above them. Placing a blind fold on the follower will add another layer to this exercise as well, leaving more room for anticipation. With this intimacy practice, only one of you will lead for the day and the other will take over the following day but if you want to exchange in that moment, then take an extra day to change leader and follower. Another variation is for the leader to lay behind the follower. Start from the head and work your way down, avoiding the genitals. Take your time to slowly build up the sensation by repeating 'Intimacy Practice 2' before working on the genital area. Both of you can also take the time to explore the chest and breast area by kissing and stroking around the breast area (more details in 'Intimacy Practice 4', page 89).

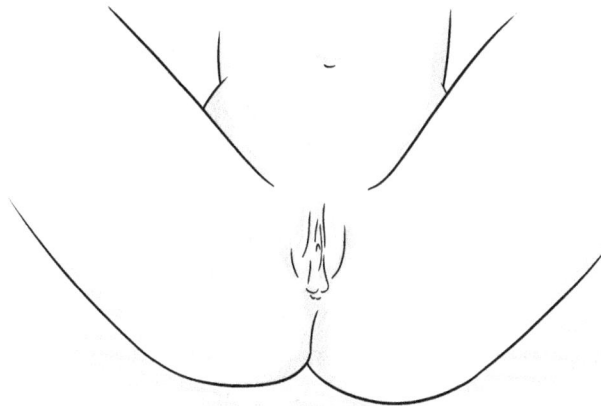

For the guys, gently spread your female partner's legs with yours by rubbing her inner thighs slowly and taking time to slowly explore the vulva. The top of the vulva is the pubic area and as you go deeper, there are the inner and outer lips, clitoris, and vagina opening. Make a circular motion around the vaginal opening, as well as extending a larger circle to include the clitoris. Some refer to this circular motion as the ring of fire that not only teases your partner but also creates a desire for you to explore the inside of her vagina. After making sure that she is properly lubricated, gently slip your finger into the front opening. Allow her to relax before going any further. You can also apply a slight pressure on her g-spot—a ridged spot located about two inches away from the opening of the vagina. Continue teasing but do not go any further until you feel her vulva swell and see that she is in an aroused state. If she is uncomfortable or prefers to guide your hand, allow her to lead your hand to her desired sweet spot.

For the ladies, take your position behind your man and work your way top-down. When exploring the penis, wrap your hand around the flaccid or erect penis and start with slight alternating pulses or pressure, while observing your partner's erection and reaction. This 'press and hold' technique is a way to simulate intercourse and will help encourage blood flow if your partner has problems achieving an erection. Another technique is to wrap your hand around the testicles and gently press or pull them down. Then check your partner's reaction to see if he enjoys the sensation. Be gentle though as some men enjoy this sensation and others do not. You can also take one hand and wrap it around the shaft of the penis with slight pressing movement while the other cradles the testicles. You can also run your fingers or tongue up and down the head of the penis where there is a v shape as well as under the head of the penis. If your partner is uncircumcised and the penis is erect, you can gently move the skin under the head of the penis so as to rub the underside of the head of the penis and expose the head.

Genital play can be a wonderful experience for couples who usually go straight into intercourse. Encouraging exploration in different ways promotes sensuality and adds new experiences to your sex notes. However, the objective of this practice is not to give your partner an orgasm, but to understand what feels pleasurable for both of you. This is done by exploring, touching, and enjoying the process of giving pleasure to yourself and your partner. That said, is it completely fine for you to masturbate in front of each other if either of you gets aroused during this practice. Own your own pleasure as well as take care of your pleasure on your own.

NOTES

NOTES

NOTES

_____

_____

_____

_____

_____

_____

_____

_____

_____

_____

NOTES

_____

_____

_____

_____

_____

_____

_____

_____

_____

_____

_____

NOTES

_____

_____

_____

_____

_____

_____

_____

_____

_____

NOTES

_____

_____

_____

_____

_____

_____

_____

_____

INTIMACY PRACTICE 4

In this practice, you and your partner will need to explore each other's genitals using both your hands and mouth. You will also learn new ways to please your partner and discover novel forms of masturbation. As with all of the practices mentioned in the earlier chapters, both you and your partner should take turns, with one initiating and the other on the receiving end. There is no pressure here to perform or reach orgasm. It will be an added bonus if you can get your partner to reach orgasm during this practice!

For the ladies, make an effort to incorporate some penis play and observe how your partner reacts to different ways of stroking his penis. Experiment with different types of pressure, as well as softer or lighter touches. One way is to stroke the penis slightly using a downward stroke where the hand is placed between your partner's stomach and the edge of his penis. Applying pressure between the scrotum and the anus or licking or rubbing this area can also stimulate the prostate and be very pleasurable for some men. You can also explore his penis and testicles with your mouth. However, this is not mandatory and should only be done when both of you are ready for oral sex. Some women have confessed that they do not want to give oral sex because they are put off by the thought of having semen in their mouths while others have found initiating oral sex to be an empowering experience where they can take charge of the session. For the uninitiated, a couple of ways to experiment with giving oral sex is to hold the base of the penis and use your hand to guide it into your mouth. The best position to do this is to have your partner sitting on the bed or a chair and for you to be on the floor with a pillow under your feet. This allows you to guide the penis in your mouth. For those who are uncomfortable with swallowing semen, one way to go around this is to have your partner ejaculate under your tongue and let it slowly drip out of your mouth. This is a technique that many porn stars use while giving oral sex.

For the gentlemen, start by kissing and touching your partner's face with your fingers or tongue, and work towards the breasts circling the nipples but not touching them. Tease her until her nipples are erect and slowly tickling the nipple with your tongue. Some women like having their nipples held in between two fingers and flicked back and forth slightly as this form of nipple play releases the feel good hormone, oxytocin. Once you have spent some time teasing and caressing her nipples, slowly work your way down to her tummy and her vulva. Once you see that

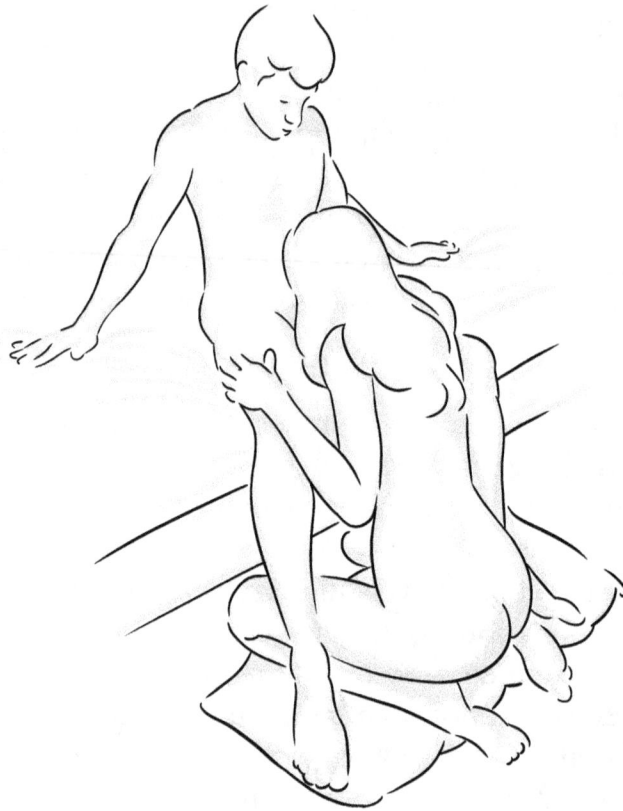

she is fully aroused, proceed to perform the ring of fire with your tongue. Start with light circular motions around the opening of the vagina and gently make your way to her clitoris. Be sure that she is aroused before touching the tip of her clitoris and take note not to overstimulate it. As mentioned in 'Positive Sex Education' on page 13, the clitoris has clitoral legs that run under the skin, into the vagina and cluster in the opening of the vagina—the G spot. Once your partner is aroused and well lubricated, put your finger in her vagina and place some pressure on the upper wall while using your tongue to gently lick around the clitoras. Some women enjoy direct clitoral stimulation while others prefer indirect clitoral stimulation, i.e. a lighter touch or pressure. Do note that her preferences will also change according to her menstrual cycle and hormones. The objective of the exercise is to find out what turns your partner on.

If you and your partner are toying with the idea of anal stimulation, this is a good opportunity to try this out. I have consulted both male and female clients who have reported having better orgasms with proper anal stimulation. Using your fingers or tongue to probe around the opening of the anus can be very pleasing for both men and women. If you decide to experiment with oral penetration, you can use your tongue and saliva to lick around the anus before slowly inserting your tongue. For finger penetration, make sure you use lubrication and start very slowly as there are two very strong muscles that are at the opening and inside of the opening of the anus, and these muscles need to be relaxed before penetration. Forcing any objects, finger or penis into the anus without it being fully relaxed can result in tearing the delicate skin around the opening. A clean bum is a must too! As with all the other intimacy practices, be constantly aware of your partner's feelings throughout the session.

NOTES

_____

_____

_____

_____

_____

_____

_____

_____

_____

Notes

_____

_____

_____

_____

_____

_____

_____

_____

_____

NOTES

NOTES

_____

_____

_____

_____

_____

_____

_____

_____

_____

_____

NOTES

_____

_____

_____

_____

_____

_____

_____

_____

_____

NOTES

INTIMACY PRACTICE 5

You are ready for 'Intimacy Practice 5', which involves the mental aspect of erotic thoughts self-pleasure and role play.

SHARING FANTASIES AND EROTIC IMAGES

Sharing fantasies and erotic images is a wonderful way for couples to be intimate. To begin this practice, spend time with your partner and talk about a fantasy that you have in details. If you have erotic images that symbolize your fantasy or a video that you have always wanted to share with your partner, this is the perfect time to do so. An interesting observation that I have made while counseling couples is that the simple act of merely talking about the fantasy can evoke emotions of thrill without even engaging in the act of the fantasy. Some people fantasize about something that they may never want to try in life but enjoy talking about with a partner. You can also take this opportunity to touch or caress your partner while sharing your fantasy. The act of talking about one's fantasy and being gently caressed at the same time can be a real turn-on.

CASE IN POINT

Bernice and Simon, a couple that I consulted was dealing with the issue of cuckolding. Simon had always secretly fantasized about being a cuckold and watching his wife have sex with other men that were more endowed than him. While he had attempted to satisfy his fetish by watching pornography videos on cuckolding, he really wanted to share this fantasy with Bernice. He finally got the courage to tell her about his fetish and this alone brought him immense satisfaction. There are also instances where a couple decides to role play a particular fantasy. Some of these include visiting a BDSM club, engaging in domination and submission acts, taking a trip to the sex store or even the simple act of purchasing sex toys together online and using them on each other.

MUTUAL SELF-PLEASURE

While most of us have pleasured ourselves sexually and know exactly what feels good, we rarely take the time to show this in person to our partner. In this exercise, you need to educate your partner on how you like pleasuring yourself and what turns you on. This can be done in either an educational, erotic, or intimate way. Encourage your partner to ask questions if needed. Sexual intimacy is about connecting, and intercourse can be wonderful for many couples when they learn how to connect through avenues other than the body and mind. When self-pleasuring, you can either use hands to demonstrate or introduce a sex toy—these are two fun ways to bring pleasure to parts of the body. You can incorporate massage, tantra, scented oils, blindfolds, feathers, and sexy lingerie. Apart from talking about your fantasy while touching yourself in front of your partner, role play and dirty talk are highly encouraged as well.

Do note that all of the above recommendations listed in this practice can be repeated until both you and your partner are ready to move on to the next practice. 'Intimacy Practice #5' is designed to allow you and your partner to explore each other's minds and bodies sexually without the pressure to perform sexually. Finding out each other's pleasure zones and fantasies is the objective of this practice. 'Intimacy Practice 5' works exceptionally well with men who have issues with erectile dysfunction or are recovering from prostate cancer, and those have other health issues such as disabilities or even PTSD. Women who are not able to achieve orgasms, experience pain during intercourse, have health issues, experience lack of desire, or or practise? suffer from other sexual issues can also benefit from this practice.

NOTES

_____

_____

_____

_____

_____

_____

_____

_____

_____

_____

NOTES

_____

_____

_____

_____

_____

_____

_____

_____

_____

_____

_____

NOTES

_____

_____

_____

_____

_____

_____

_____

_____

_____

NOTES

NOTES

_____

_____

_____

_____

_____

_____

_____

_____

_____

NOTES

_____

_____

_____

_____

_____

_____

_____

_____

_____

INTIMACY PRACTICE 6

Congratulations! You and your partner have breezed through all five intimacy practices. The final practice in this series focuses on the pleasure of intercourse and includes a variety of fun positions to explore.

Often times, couples will fall into a routine or pattern and on average, most couples will keep to one or two positions without being aware that their love life can benefit from incorporating a variety of positions. Women are capable of experiencing amazing orgasms as well as multiple orgasms though different positions and variations of stimulation. In addition, the act of intercourse can be a way to emotionally and physically connect on a much deeper level. For a woman, allowing a trusted partner to enter one's body can be a wonderfully emotional and enjoyable experience. Often times, the best position for achieving orgasm during intercourse is when she can control the intensity of the penetration. As such, positions associated with her being on top or on her side so that she can control the depth and speed of intercourse are ideal. This angle also provides clitoral stimulation as the penis rubs again it during penetration. If your partner enjoys this position, you can

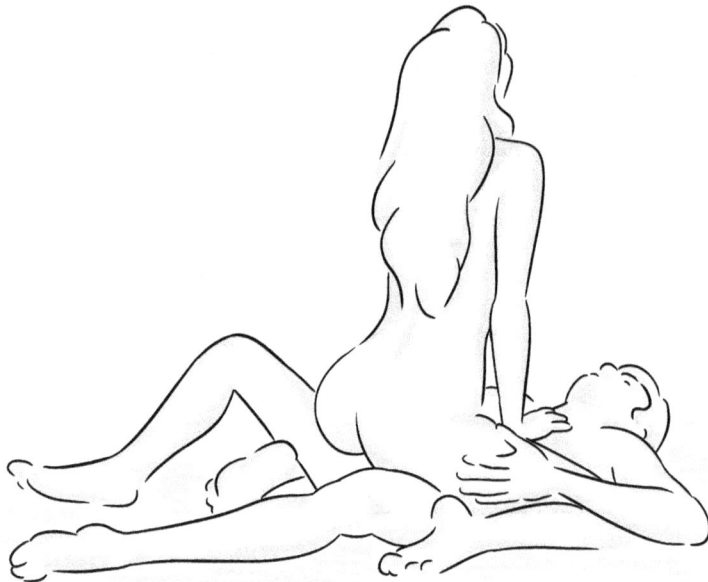

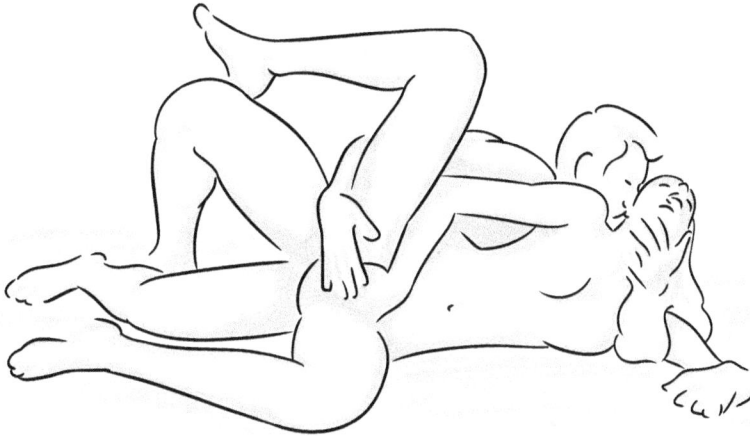

take this opportunity to relax and take in the magnificent view of her pleasing her-self with your penis. You can also kiss her at the same time or play with her breasts and nipples as she literally rocks your world. For the ladies, you can begin this posi-tion with a huge teaser—only penetrating the opening and first two inches of your vagina and rubbing his penis against your g-spot.

Another recommended position is for the man to enter his partner from the side because she can then ease his penis in and sling her leg over him easily while he stimulates her clitoris with his fingers. This also allows him access to her neck and he can further tease her with kisses along this erogenous zone. She can also reach down and stimulate the penis during penetration at the same time and reach around to stroke the testicles. This position works especially well for men who are struggling with early ejaculation. Another sexy wonderful advantage of this position is you and your partner can continue to cuddle each other or even have a pleasure nap in this position even after sex.

Enjoying the process of lovemaking by experimenting and trying new positions can add bring passion back into the sexual experience. Take turns exploring, giving and receiving pleasure and be patience with each other's needs. Below are six more of my favorite positions that have proved to maintain a longer and more passionate love making session.

ROCKING HORSE

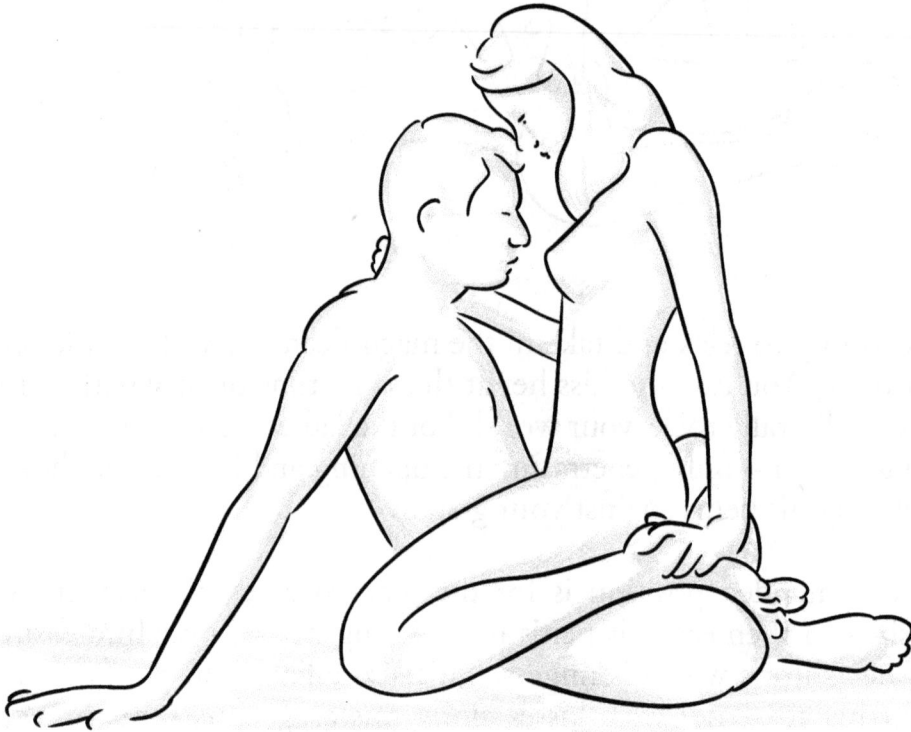

This is a wonderful position because the you and your partner can face each other. This allows kissing and slow passionate penetration to take place. In this position, the man sits cross-legged and leans back by supporting himself with both arms behind him or leaning against a wall. The woman then kneels over his lap, hugs him with her thighs and lowers herself down at the speed and depth that she determines. This also allows her to adjust her position for clitoral stimulation.

THE CURLED ANGEL (AKA ANJOU-STYLE)

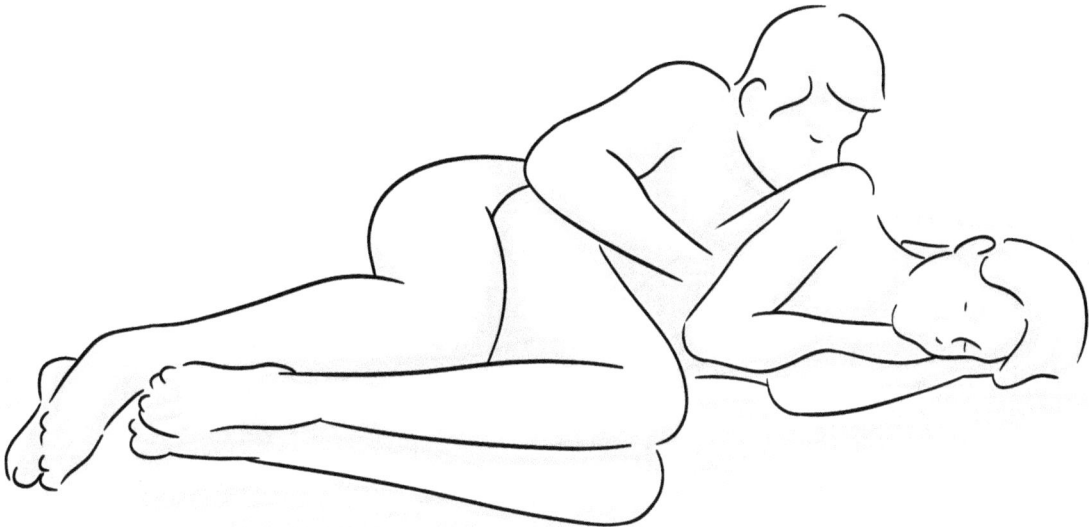

In this position, the woman curls up on her side with her knees drawn up and the man spoons her from behind. Penetration is fairly easy and the man can reach around to touch her breast and clitoris. This position is also good for deep penetration that can be done in a slower motion while still maintaining an embrace. This is a wonderful position for women who are pregnant. The man can cuddle her, kiss her neck, ear and face while slowly and intimately making love at the same time.

GLOWING JUNIPER

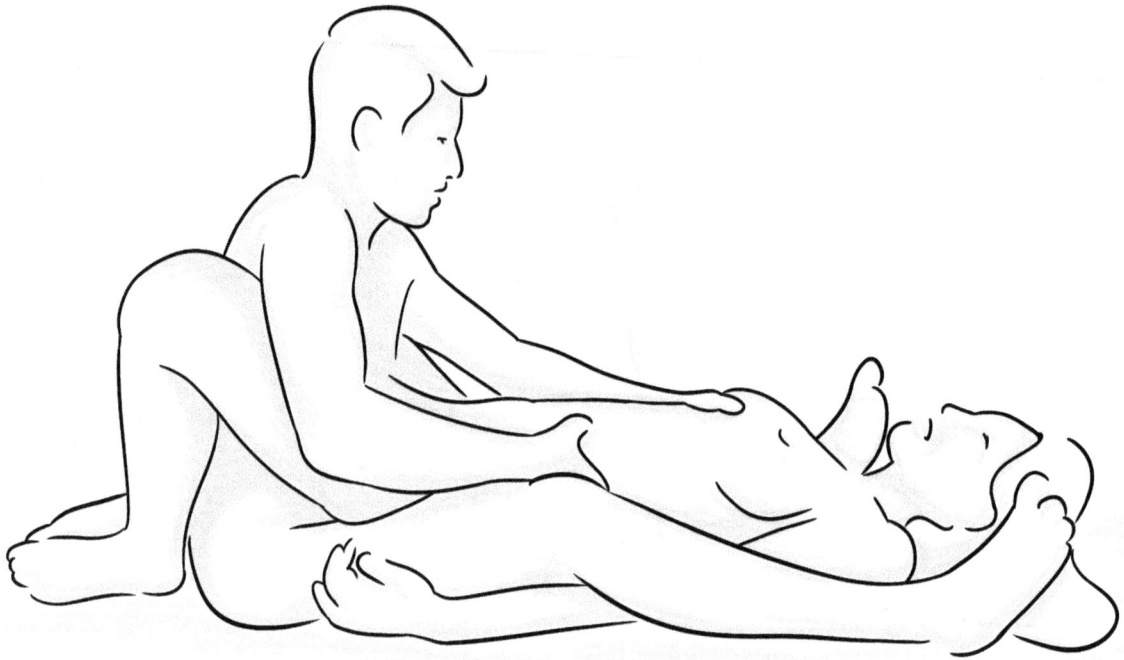

In this position, the woman lies on her back with her legs open and outstretched. The man then sits between her knees and faces her with his legs outstretched. He can lean against a wall or pillow for more comfort. This is a position that provides flexibility as he has the option of lifting her hips to aid penetration while leaning down to kiss her belly, breasts and face at the same time. This is a romantic position favoured by many couples.

Rowing boat

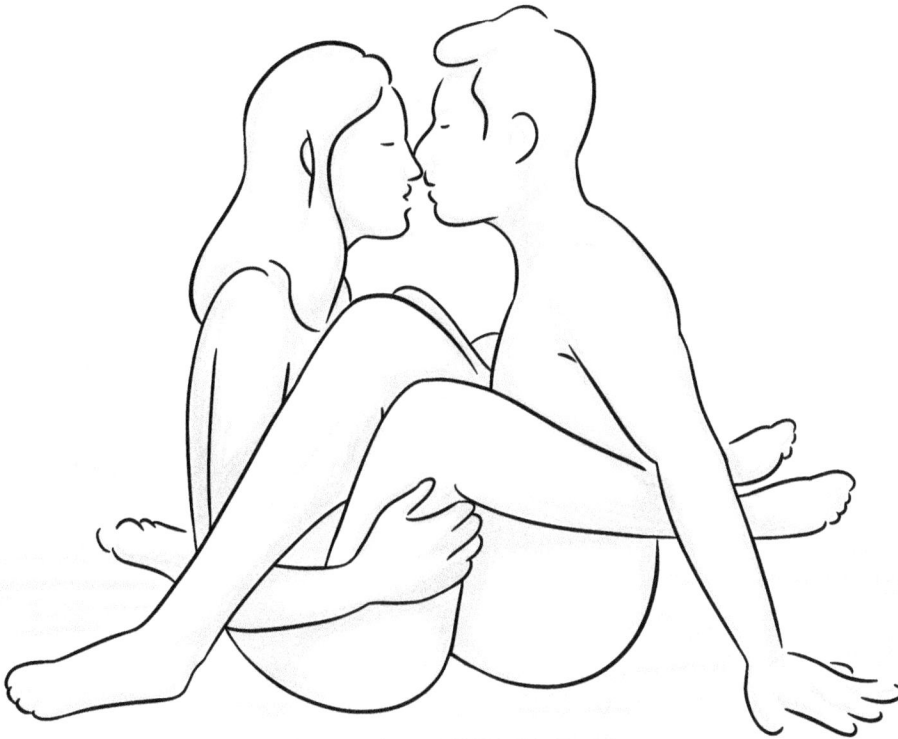

To get into this position, the man starts by lying back so the woman can sit down slowly on to his penis. The man then sits up, bringing his knees and torso up so that both the couple is face to face and his knees are placed around of her body. She should also have her knees bent up so her legs are outside his and she can wrap her legs around him. He then slips his arms over her calves and under her knees and she slips her hands under his knees and round her thighs so that she can grip his hands to form the rocking position. This is an intimate position where you and your partner are face to face, looking in each other's eyes. The position involves slow penetration and you can both rock your bodies together to create the thrusting motion.

THE PEG

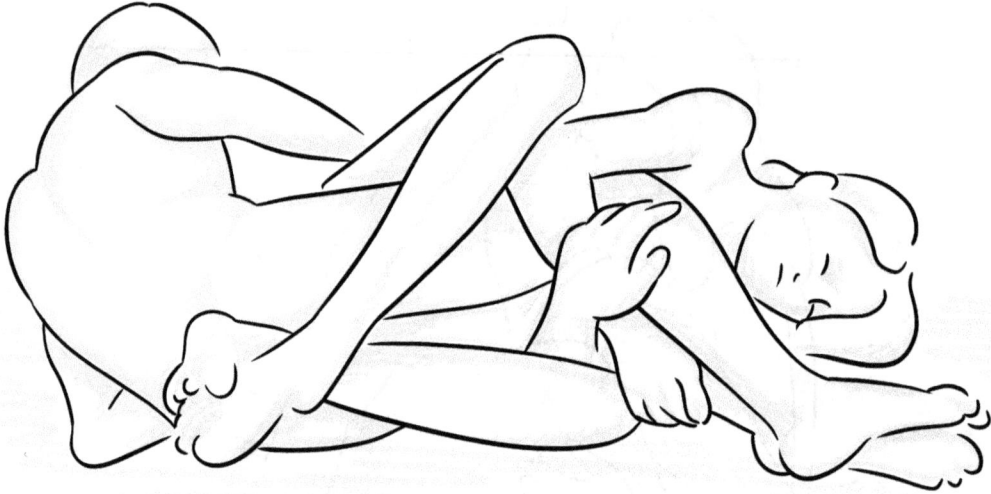

In this position, the man lies down on his back with his legs stretched out. The woman then gets on top of him and lets him enter her. As he does so, she stretches her legs out straight behind her and starts to move back and forth according to her desire. This position allows full body contact, kissing and touching throughout. When her legs are placed together, this creates a tighter fit for the couple during penetration. The intimacy of having the woman lying on top of the man and being able to hug each other while having slow long thrusting penetration is the highlight of this position.

Now, pick a few of these positions that both you and your partner like and try them out. Remember that having intimate sex is a process and once you get to the last chapter of this guidebook, it is recommended for the both of you to revisit the practices again. Make sure to jot down some of your experiences as a reference and check in on your progress at least once every three months. Research has shown that it takes about three months to fully adopt new habits and this includes embracing the habit of intimate sex too. In addition, make an effort to be proactive in your relationship. Great sex does not just happen and it takes two to keep the passion burning.

Everyone deserves to have a healthy sex life, and so do you!

NOTES

_____

_____

_____

_____

_____

_____

_____

_____

_____

NOTES

NOTES

_____

_____

_____

_____

_____

_____

_____

_____

_____

NOTES

NOTES

_____

_____

_____

_____

_____

_____

_____

_____

_____

_____

_____

NOTES

_____

_____

_____

_____

_____

_____

_____

_____

_____

[ELEVEN]

DATE NIGHT

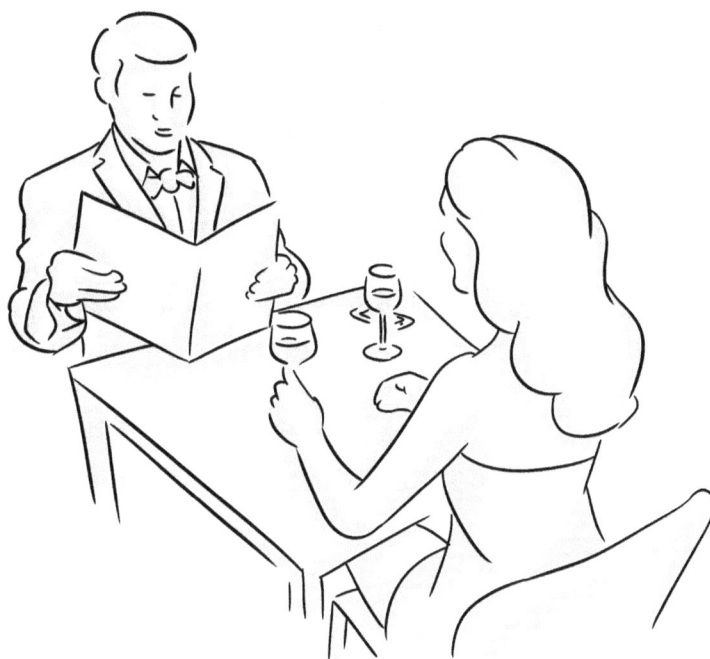

HAVING a date night once a week or at least twice a month is an important aspect of maintaining the intimacy outside the bedroom. The rules for date night are as follows:

1. Talk about anything but the kids, work, or stressors
2. Keep it fun, and talk about future plans or things you have in common.
3. Try out a new restaurant, get adventurous and visit a sex shop, or shop online for some sexy lingerie after you get home from a night out.

The idea is to spend quality time with each other and constantly come up with new ideas of potential places to go to or activities to try out together. When planning the date night or even a short vacation, both parties should take turns planning. This removes the pressure on one to always be responsible for coming up or arranging the date and ensures that both parties are responsible for working on the relationship.

It may take three months for a pattern to be established. Hence, it is highly recommended for you and your partner to refer to this guide every six months as a refresher and to add new ideas to the list. It is also best that the both of you make time to complete the entire set of exercises together once a week and use brainstorm on novel date night ideas at least a month in advance. You should also take turns and attempt to add a new event or activity that you would like the other to try out. Last but not least, make an effort to spend at least once every month doing what your partner likes and take turns to introduce them to activities that you are interested in. This is a great way to show the commitment to be with each other in a relationship. Some couples have found that after they having taken the initiative to try something out new, both of them ended up having more common interests and this further strengthens the bond.

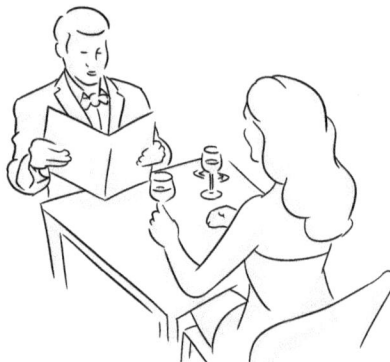

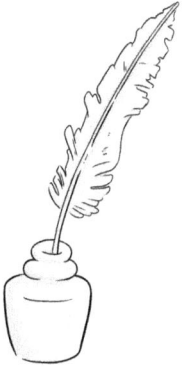

DATE NIGHT ACTIVITY PLANNER

1)

2)

3)

4)

5)

6)

7)

8)

9)

10)

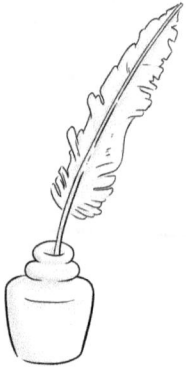

DATE NIGHT ACTIVITY PLANNER

1)

2)

3)

4)

5)

6)

7)

8)

9)

10)

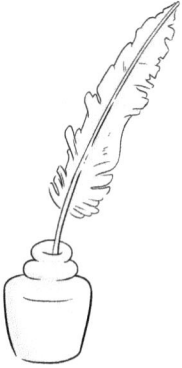

DATE NIGHT ACTIVITY PLANNER

1)

2)

3)

4)

5)

6)

7)

8)

9)

10)

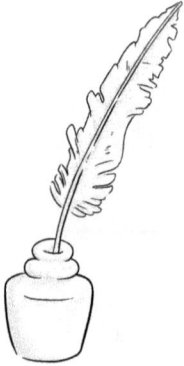

DATE NIGHT ACTIVITY PLANNER

1)

2)

3)

4)

5)

6)

7)

8)

9)

10)

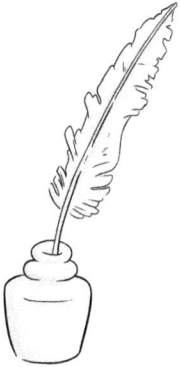

Date Night Activity Planner

1)

2)

3)

4)

5)

6)

7)

8)

9)

10)

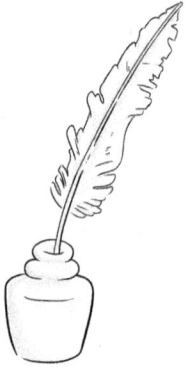

DATE NIGHT ACTIVITY PLANNER

1)

2)

3)

4)

5)

6)

7)

8)

9)

10)

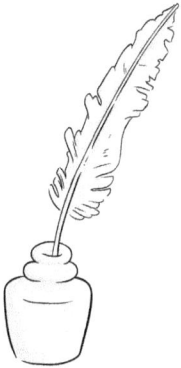

LIST OF PLACES WE BOTH ENJOY GOING TOGETHER

1)

2)

3)

4)

5)

6)

7)

8)

9)

10)

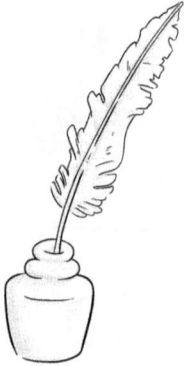

List of Places We Both Enjoy Going Together

1)

2)

3)

4)

5)

6)

7)

8)

9)

10)

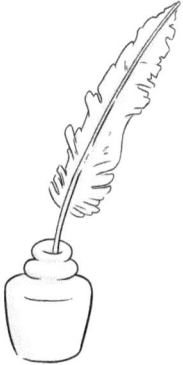

LIST OF PLACES WE BOTH ENJOY GOING TOGETHER

1)

2)

3)

4)

5)

6)

7)

8)

9)

10)

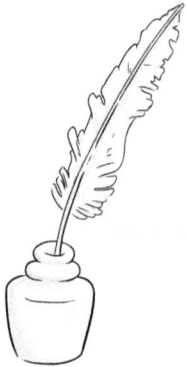

LIST OF PLACES WE BOTH ENJOY GOING TOGETHER

1)

2)

3)

4)

5)

6)

7)

8)

9)

10)

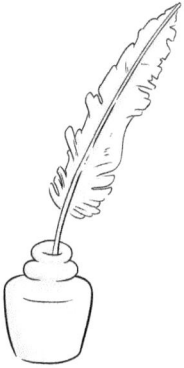

LIST OF PLACES WE BOTH ENJOY GOING TOGETHER

1)

2)

3)

4)

5)

6)

7)

8)

9)

10)

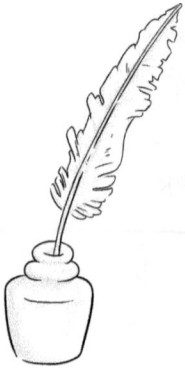

LIST OF PLACES WE BOTH ENJOY GOING TOGETHER

1)

2)

3)

4)

5)

6)

7)

8)

9)

10)

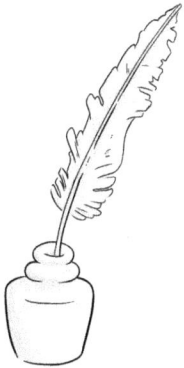

LIST OF PLACES WE BOTH ENJOY GOING TOGETHER

1)

2)

3)

4)

5)

6)

7)

8)

9)

10)

CONCLUSION

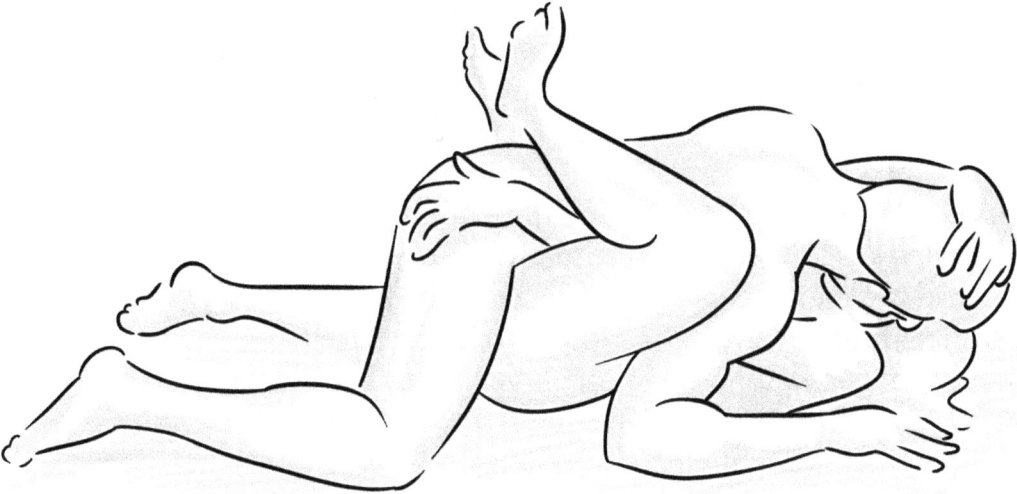

JENNIFER and Mark are a very adorable couple who arranged for an appointment at my office because they wanted to spice up their sex life. They have been married for more than 20 years and while they loved each other and were still very much attracted to each other, their sex life had become a routine and they wanted to add some intimacy and fun back into it. They were in their 40s, obviously still very much in love and they wanted to make sure that they would still have the passion for each other in the many more years to come. I worked with this wonderful couple for six sessions and could see how with each session, they were opening up to each other in new ways while having fun trying novel activities together.

After the last session, Jennifer and Mark came to my office and shared their experience. Mark then talked about the special evening that Jennifer had planned for him the night before. As recommended in this guidebook, it was Jennifer's turn to initiate the session and she had bought some new sexy lingerie. The idea was for her to take over and create her own sexy scene. She asked Mark to sit in a chair before walking into the room in her sexy outfit and teased him throughout, telling him he could only look at her until she was ready to touch him. Jennifer then made him place his hands behind his back and she used her body and lips to caress him all over and took it upon herself to orally stimulate him while forbidding him to move. As Mark was recalling the night, Jennifer was listening shyly with a smile on her face as it was the very first time that she had taken on the dominate role in the bedroom. She then confessed that as she was turning him on, she was getting turned on herself. She eventually allowed him to free his hands so that he could touch her as per her instructions. Jennifer also shared that she found the exchange of power in initiating and pleasing him both exciting and enjoyable. Mark then added that the following in his own words:

> *I turned to watch my wife walk back to the bathroom in her sexy outfit and the outline of her back and just how beautiful she was, her hair falling down her back and I just looked at her and said to myself that is my wife … Wow! That is my beautiful wife!*

The look of love and passion on his face was so moving that all three of us ended up crying. It was clear that Jennifer and Mark have now achieved what many of us will deem the 'impossible' in a 20-year marriage, and entered a new chapter of their lives—one filled with friendship, partnership, love, passion and deep intimacy! As a clinical sexologist and intimacy counselor, I am extremely honored that couples such Jennifer and Mark have opened up to me and allowed me to help them to create a deep connection with their sex lives. Now, take this journey with me to ignite the passion and show the commitment that they have for your partner!

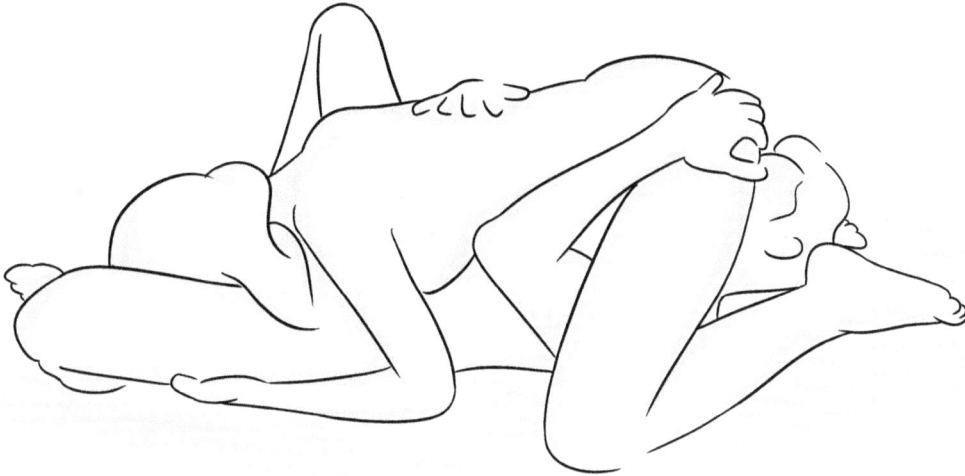

www.ingramcontent.com/pod-product-compliance
Lightning Source LLC
Chambersburg PA
CBHW052113020426
42335CB00021B/2744